The Chronic Fatigue Syndrome Mastery Bible: Your Blueprint for Complete Chronic Fatigue Syndrome Management

Dr. Ankita Kashyap and Prof. Krishna N. Sharma

Published by Virtued Press, 2023.

While every precaution has been taken in the preparation of this book, the publisher assumes no responsibility for errors or omissions, or for damages resulting from the use of the information contained herein.

THE CHRONIC FATIGUE SYNDROME MASTERY BIBLE: YOUR BLUEPRINT FOR COMPLETE CHRONIC FATIGUE SYNDROME MANAGEMENT

First edition. December 3, 2023.

ISBN: 979-8223910015

Written by Dr. Ankita Kashyap and Prof. Krishna N. Sharma.

Table of Contents

DISCLAIMER

The information provided in this book is intended for general informational purposes only. The content is not meant to substitute professional medical advice, diagnosis, or treatment. Always consult with a qualified healthcare provider before making any changes to your management plan or healthcare regimen.

While every effort has been made to ensure the accuracy and completeness of the information presented, the author and publisher do not assume any responsibility for errors, omissions, or potential misinterpretations of the content. Individual responses to management strategies may vary, and what works for one person might not be suitable for another.

The book does not endorse any specific medical treatments, products, or services. Readers are encouraged to seek guidance from their healthcare providers to determine the most appropriate approaches for their unique medical conditions and needs.

Any external links or resources provided in the book are for convenience and informational purposes only. The author and publisher do not have control over the content or availability of these external sources and do not endorse or guarantee the accuracy of such information.

Readers are advised to exercise caution and use their judgment when applying the information provided in this book to their own situations. The author and publisher disclaim any liability for any direct, indirect, consequential, or other damages arising from the use of this book and its content.

By reading and using this book, readers acknowledge and accept the limitations and inherent risks associated with implementing the strategies, recommendations, and information contained herein. It is always recommended to consult a qualified healthcare professional for personalized medical advice and care.

Introduction

I am a lighthouse of holistic healthcare in the maze of contemporary medicine, when patients frequently feel like little more than symptoms. In addition to practising medicine, I am a passionate health and wellness coach who is dedicated to the complete field of healing arts and sciences. My name is Dr. Ankita Kashyap. My hands have planted the soil of wellness and written prescriptions with equal ease throughout the years; the journeys of each patient bear witness to this symbiotic dance between science and spirit.

The strict underpinnings of traditional medicine set the stage for my journey through the medical landscape, which culminated in a thriving practise where integrating complementary approaches is not an afterthought but the cornerstone of our approach. In the mosaic of recovery, I came onto Chronic Fatigue Syndrome (CFS) as a persistent mystery that casts doubt on the vitality of the human soul.

The honours that surround my name, from academic publications to the moving testimonies of people I've assisted, are not trinkets; rather, they are the reflections of lives that have been impacted and changed. They are the validation of innumerable hours devoted to comprehending not only the "what" of CFS but also the "why" and "how" of its mastery.

I am sharing this storey from the trenches of personal investment rather than from an ivory tower of medical jargon. I've held the hands of tired people in my clinic and witnessed their desperation in their eyes as they begged for more than a little break. "The Chronic Fatigue Syndrome Mastery Bible" emerged from this compassionate crucible, serving not just as an informational guide but also as a lifeline for those who are extremely exhausted, with each word holding the promise of hope.

Let me now invite you into a world in which having CFS is merely an illness that has to be managed rather than a life sentence. This well-researched and beautifully written book serves as your guide to managing Chronic Fatigue Syndrome holistically. You will explore the most recent findings in science and medicine with every page, all presented in language that both educates and uplifts the reader.

Have you ever been so overwhelmed by the medical jargon and the intricacies of your condition? Here, we eliminate the complexity in favour of simplicity and clarity. These sections provide methods and plans that may be customised to fit your own storey, so the advice you discover here is not only pertinent but also resonates with your own requirements.

Imagine living a life where dealing with CFS is a shared experience rather than a lonely battle. Imagine a road map that blends the gentle force of dietary planning, lifestyle adjustments, and psychological support with the accuracy of medical care. Imagine adopting self-help methods that give you the ability to take back control of your life and reduce symptoms at the same time.

The path to mastery for Chronic Fatigue Syndrome is, in fact, extremely specific to you and your battle with it. This book is your guide; it's accommodating and perceptive, willing to change to suit your needs as you go. Every tactic and piece of advise given here is intended to meet you where you are and help you reach your goals.

With so many voices vying for your attention, you might be wondering why you should listen to this one. The answer is found in the unwavering dedication to evidence-based insights, the well-balanced integration of holistic and medical viewpoints, and the assurance that your journey is precious here.

Instead of a one-size-fits-all strategy, these pages offer a range of options that are just ready to be customised to match the unique circumstances of your life. This book is a tapestry woven with the threads of holistic care, covering everything from the science of nutrition to the art of mindfulness, the fundamentals of exercise to the haven of sleep.

Recall that mastery is a process and an ongoing unfolding, not a destination, as we set out on this adventure together. With "The Chronic Fatigue Syndrome Mastery Bible," you hold not just a book but also a lighthouse that shines on the way to a life that is defined by potential waiting to be realised rather than by weariness.

Thus, my dear reader, let me extend my hand to you. Together, let us traverse this route. As we turn each page, let's hope for a fresh start, a step toward mastering your vitality and a chapter toward the life you deserve. Here is your guide to managing Chronic Fatigue Syndrome from start to finish. Greetings from empowerment. Greetings from hope.

Understanding Chronic Fatigue Syndrome

Defining Chronic Fatigue Syndrome

Understanding is the key to managing and recovering from the complex road towards health and well-being. I beg you to stop and think about the map, the terminology that will make sense of this complicated maze and help you find your way. Because in the absence of these, we can find ourselves aimlessly wandering.

Myalgic encephalomyelitis (ME), another name for Chronic Fatigue Syndrome (CFS), is a mystery that has puzzled doctors for many years. Imagine having to bargain with your body just to get out of bed in the morning because the weight is so great that every step feels like a Herculean effort. Individuals with CFS have to deal with this on a daily basis.

It is essential to understand that CFS is more than just "feeling weary." Past the debilitating exhaustion, a range of symptoms may manifest, such as cognitive deficits, sleep deprivation, and an unusual condition called Post-Exertional Malaise (PEM). PEM, the defining feature of CFS, is an unequal and frequently delayed surge in energy that occurs after even mild physical or mental exertion. It can be likened to a cell phone that runs out of battery life after a short call and takes an excessive amount of time to recharge.

Making a diagnosis is a painstaking procedure that involves assembling a jigsaw out of a variety of symptoms that defiantly refuse to fit neatly into the parameters of conventional medical testing. The diagnostic criteria have changed throughout time, but they always centre around one thing: severe, inexplicable exhaustion that lasts longer than six months and is not brought on by continuous activity or markedly alleviated by rest.

Why is this relevant? Imagine living a life where everyday chores seem impossible and are obscured by fog. CFS is more than just a bother; it's a disorder that can turn the colourful spectrum of life into a grayscale of tiredness. By providing definitions for these phrases, we help people understand and manage this complex disease by validating the experience and acknowledging the struggle.

Have you ever been so exhausted from a long day that you just wanted to curl up in bed? Now multiply it ten times and picture a world without respite or post-rest recuperation. This is the constant exhaustion that people with CFS go through. It is a profound, pervasive exhaustion that permeates every cell and mind, and it is radically different from the weariness that the normal person experiences.

However, what does it actually mean to have CFS? It steals milestones and moments, and for many, it is a thief. It is an unseen enemy that requires a change in one's way of living, working, and engaging with the outside world. Resilience, however, is exhibited by this obstacle, demonstrating the strength of the human spirit even in the face of extreme exhaustion.

In the upcoming chapters, we will delve deeper into the complexities of CFS, examining the scientific foundations, the disputes, and the firsthand accounts of those who experience this condition. Since knowledge is our most powerful tool against the stigma and misunderstandings, we shall empower ourselves with it.

As we approach the start of this trip, I want to know what it means to really listen to your body. To follow its cues, even if they require a complete stop? Chronic fatigue syndrome is not only a disease; it is a mentor, teaching us about the limits of human potential and the importance of equilibrium.

Let's keep in mind that even while CFS may be chronic, a person's life does not have to be defined by it. Let's construct a tapestry of empathy and understanding with every word we read because understanding fosters hope. Even though the journey will be lengthy and the weight heavy, we will go across this terrain together, turning hardship into advocacy and exhaustion into strength.

The Symptoms Spectrum

Recognizing the symptoms of Chronic Fatigue Syndrome is the first step towards comprehending the condition, just as the sun's warm fingers signifying the beginning of a new day. The condition is represented by a tapestry made of threads with different colours and thicknesses, each of which symbolises a different manifestation of Chronic Fatigue Syndrome (CFS). Understanding the range of symptoms is crucial, reader, since it holds the key to gaining control of CFS and enabling efficient management.

Permit me to briefly describe what lies ahead of us before we dive into the core of these manifestations. We will discuss the primary symptoms that make up the CFS constellation as well as the more subdued, less obvious symptoms that frequently go unrecognised but are extremely important to the everyday lives of those who are impacted. Knowing this spectrum can help people who are lost in the sea of doubt that CFS can produce; it is more than just an academic exercise.

Our exploration will take us through:
- Profound Fatigue
- Cognitive Impairments
- Sleep Abnormalities
- Orthostatic Intolerance
- Pain and Sensitivity
- Neurological Oddities
- Immune System Irregularities
- Gastrointestinal Disturbances
- Emotional and Psychological Impact

Overwhelming exhaustion that is unaffected by rest and out of proportion to any effort is the defining feature of CFS. Fatigue casts a relentless shadow that obscures even the most routine everyday duties. Patients frequently describe it as feeling like they are wading through molasses, needing to exert enormous effort with every step.

CFS causes mental fog. Slow processing speeds, memory lapses, and concentration issues can all be signs of this "brain fog." Envision a computer that is inundated with an excessive number of tasks, causing each application to launch more slowly and eventually causing the system to crash.

For many with CFS, sleep turns from being a place of rejuvenation to a perverse irony. Patients may experience insomnia or unrefreshing sleep in spite of their weariness. Sleep is seen but not felt, like when you're parched and there's a glass of water just out of reach.

Orthostatic intolerance is the term for the dizzying drop in blood pressure that many CFS patients experience when they stand up. This can have the sensation of an unkind game of gravity, where getting up too fast could result in a faint dance or a fall to the ground.

Pain is not avoided by CFS patients. Patients may experience constant pain in their muscles and joints as well as increased sensitivity to light, sound, and touch—a world in which even the slightest contact from a piece of cloth can feel like sandpaper on the skin.

CFS causes a bewildering assortment of neurological symptoms, ranging from pins and needles to migraines. The body may appear to be malfunctioning, sending out signals of pain and discomfort for no apparent reason.

The symptoms of the immune system might be paradoxical, exhibiting both overreactivity and underperformance. Patients may struggle with a persistent feeling of being "under the weather" or become caught in a cycle of recurring infections.

An intestinal revolt brought on by CFS frequently results in nausea, bloating, and a variety of bowel problems. One must constantly bargain with their own body, maintaining a fine equilibrium that is easily thrown off.

There is more to CFS than just physical weight. It has an emotional cost that strains mental health by causing worry, irritation, and feelings of loneliness. It's a darkness that touches the core of a person's being and reaches beyond their outward manifestations.

Every symptom is a part of a chorus, with each voice blending into the next, rather than an isolated experience. Not only is there evidence for these symptoms in medical literature, but the experiences of people with CFS also bear witness to them. Each of their testimonies attests to the intricacy of this disease, as they describe the unwavering quest for normalcy among the clamour of symptoms.

Recognizing the range of symptoms is really the beginning; it is not the end. It provides guidance for customised methods in holistic therapy, nutrition, coping mechanisms, and lifestyle adjustments. To ease gastrointestinal issues, for example, food planning might emphasise gut health; to ease the body back into activity without aggravating exhaustion, graded exercise could be introduced.

Transitions through the Spectrum

Always keep in mind that every patient's experience with CFS is as distinct as their fingerprint as we work through the symptoms. One can be more affected by cognitive decline, while another might be trapped in excruciating discomfort. It is our responsibility to comprehend the intricate dance of intertwined symptoms.

You may wonder why this spectrum is so important to our path. For to treat CFS, my dear reader, is to comprehend it—not just in the clinical sense, but also in the lived reality of individuals who suffer from it. Each symptom has layers that can be peeled back to reveal chances for intervention, support, and hope.

Let's conclude with some empowerment. Now that we know more, we can better attack the mystery of CFS. We are able to navigate through the storm of symptoms and arrive at the more tranquil waters of health and energy. This is our goal, our road map to success, and we will travel it together with poise and resolve.

Historical Perspective on CFS

Have you ever wondered how doctors of the past viewed the illnesses we deal with today? The history of Chronic Fatigue Syndrome (CFS), a complicated and frequently misdiagnosed illness, has been especially mysterious. Let's explore the history of CFS and follow its footsteps across the ephemeral sands of time.

Neurasthenia, a name coined by American neurologist George Beard, was used in the 1800s to describe a disorder that had striking similarities to what is now known as CFS. Headaches, exhaustion, and a host of other symptoms typified the malaise of the times. Was it, however, the same as the CFS that exists today? Understanding patterns show up as we unravel the wide and varied historical tapestry.

The important turning points in the diagnosis and research of CFS happened in a chronological dance with medical advancements. In the 20th century, there was a notable outbreak at Los Angeles County Hospital in 1934. At first, poliomyelitis was suspected, but because of its distinct appearance, poliomyelitis was eventually reclassified as "atypical poliomyelitis." This was possibly one of the first cases of a condition similar to CFS that was documented.

Over time, comparable outbreaks in different places—like the Royal Free Hospital in London in 1955—have increased the suspicion of a novel, separate condition. Every occurrence functioned as a puzzle piece, gradually creating a picture of a state that eluded simple classification.

Imagine, if you will, the multicoloured threads that make up the global CFS tapestry. The term "myalgic encephalomyelitis" (ME) was coined in the UK to emphasise the pain in the muscles and the possible inflammation of the brain and spinal cord. The United States, on the other hand, preferred "Chronic Fatigue Syndrome," emphasising continuous tiredness that was not eased by rest. These cultural distinctions in naming highlighted differing viewpoints on genesis and disease in addition to linguistic differences.

CFS came to prominence in the 1980s and 1990s as sufferers and advocacy groups pushed for acceptance from a medical community that frequently treated their condition with suspicion. Was this a case of contemporary hysteria or a real, organic illness?

The intricacy of CFS has been acknowledged by the medical profession, leading to changes in current interpretations. Though much is still unknown, scientific advances have shown possible immunological and neurological foundations. I have personal experience with the contemporary struggle for self-validation and practical coping mechanisms as a health and wellness coach.

However, there have been many difficulties and disagreements along the way to understanding CFS. The Centers for Disease Control and Prevention (CDC) case definition from 1994, which provided established diagnostic criteria for CFS, marked a turning point. There are still differences, though, with some academics and supporters calling for a redefining that more accurately reflects the intensity and range of symptoms.

What effect does this have on us now, then? Our approach to understanding CFS is being shaped by patient experiences and emerging research. We are searching for a way that will bring relief and well-being to people who are suffering, and we find ourselves at a crossroads between the shadows of the past and the promise of the future.

My method, which combines holistic health techniques with lifestyle adjustments, is proof of the contemporary rethinking of CFS treatment. It embraces the possibilities of integrative medicine while acknowledging the limitations of our historical perspective.

We have seen the transformation of CFS from an unclear illness to a recognised medical diagnosis during our journey through time. This voyage is a tapestry of human experience, woven with the threads of suffering, resiliency, and hope, rather than just a record of events. As we come to the end of this chapter, let us remember the lessons learned from the past and be determined to create a future in which the mystery surrounding CFS is dispelled by knowledge and kind treatment.

As we move forward, we remember those who have struggled with CFS and renew our commitment to a society in which no one has to face the maze of chronic illness alone. In "The Chronic Fatigue Syndrome Mastery Bible: Your Blueprint for Complete Chronic Fatigue Syndrome Management," I, Dr. Ankita Kashyap, invite you to join me as we pursue this goal.

Physiological Underpinnings

Within the stillness of our own bodies rests a symphony of processes that are harmonious when well and discordant when not. The symptoms of Chronic Fatigue Syndrome (CFS), a disorder that has long defied the full scope of medical knowledge, are so diverse that they confound scientists and patients alike. We aim to shed light on the physiological foundations of this bewildering illness in order to illuminate the murky field of CFS research.

The primary hypothesis of our investigation is that Chronic Fatigue Syndrome is a complicated condition with distinct physiological anomalies and alterations rather than just a state of weariness. This claim invites us to look past the outward signs and symptoms and investigate the cellular and systemic orchestra that highlights this illness.

The first piece of evidence we find is immunological dysfunction. A heightened immunological response is common in CFS patients, as if their bodies are constantly on the verge of infection. These people often have elevated levels of inflammatory markers, those biochemical flare guns that communicate distress, which creates an impression of internal conflict in the absence of an obvious enemy.

Further investigation reveals that this is a chronic immune condition rather than a transient immunological conflict. Patients with chronic fatigue syndrome frequently have reduced function of their natural killer cells, the body's own guardians against infections. This compromised immune system may contribute to both the early onset and the chronic character of CFS.

However, when we provide these pieces of data, counterarguments hint at the variety found in CFS cases. Certain patients do not exhibit these immunological disparities; a few even seem to have astonishingly normal immune profiles. How is it possible for a same diagnosis to have such variation?

As a result, we have to acknowledge that CFS exhibits a variety of physiological profiles, much like a chameleon. The activity of the immune system can just be one painting in a gallery of other illnesses. Moreover, not all abnormalities are immediately noticeable or consistent across many studies and groups due to the complexity of immune function and evaluation.

Delving deeper into the physiological maze, we come across indications of abnormalities in the nervous system. According to research on brain imaging, individuals with CFS frequently have smaller volumes of their white and grey matter. This is consistent with the cognitive problems that many patients describe, suggesting that the basic organisation of their brain circuits has been disrupted.

We need to pay attention to the murmurs of scepticism as we observe these changes in the brain. Are these changes just incidental effects of the lifestyle modifications brought about by chronic illness? Longitudinal studies that show the development of these anomalies, pointing to a direct association with the condition rather than a result of depression or inactivity, provide evidence against such uncertainty.

The body's currency of vitality, energy metabolism, is another area compromised by malfunction in CFS. Studies have revealed a unique metabolic profile in people with CFS; the energy factories of the cell, the mitochondria, appear to function frugally, generating energy at a sparse pace. It is as though the body has entered an unjustified and inflexible state of energy conservation.

Despite its allure, this metabolic economy is not without its detractors. Some contend that this metabolic change may have its origins in less physical activity. However, when we take into account the existence of post-exertional malaise, a defining feature of CFS in which symptoms worsen after even mild exercise, it is evident that the metabolic disruption comes before and foretells the physical restrictions, not the other way around.

In our quest for information, we also need to take into consideration the autonomic nervous system, which in CFS patients appears to have lost its steady hand in controlling physiological processes. An uncontrollable heart rate, blood pressure, and digestion can resemble a conductor who has lost control of the orchestra. This dysautonomia serves as additional evidence of the intricate physiological basis of CFS.

Upon combining the various pieces of data, we are left with a complex picture of interconnected immunological, neurological, metabolic, and autonomic dysfunctions. Every thread is essential and provides a clue to the mystery surrounding chronic fatigue syndrome.

In conclusion, there is increasing evidence to support the claim that unique physiological alterations are a hallmark of CFS, making the claim both plausible and well-founded. The claim is supported by a body of research that includes immunological abnormalities, changes in brain anatomy, metabolic shifts, and autonomic dysregulation. We can start to solve the intricate puzzle of CFS and, in the end, create a management plan by comprehending these physiological foundations.

We are reminded that the search for knowledge is about more than just the answers we discover; this is especially true as we close the book on the current chapter of our understanding. What fresh understandings will the upcoming study chapter provide? How can we develop more effective, individualised treatments based on our growing understanding of the physiological causes of CFS? These inquiries encourage us to keep going and gain control over Chronic Fatigue Syndrome. And for the benefit of everyone who yearns to regain their health and energy, we shall proceed on this crucial path with an unwavering spirit of inquiry.

Psychological Aspects of CFS

Discovering the Mind's Labyrinth in Chronic Fatigue Syndrome

Chronic fatigue syndrome, or CFS, is a journey that goes beyond the physical. As we explore the mysterious world of chronic illness, we come to understand that the mind is an integral partner in this endurance dance, just as the body is not the only one carrying the weight. When examining the complex relationship between health and sickness, the psychological components of CFS frequently take centre stage. It's a storey that develops from deep inside the mind, woven together with thought, feeling, and perception patterns that are just as significant and genuine as any physical ailment.

With all the weight of medical knowledge and compassionate insight behind me, I make the following claim: individuals with CFS experience a profound and complex psychological effect that affects their mental health and general well-being in ways that require our attention and comprehension.

The initial evidence for this notion appears in the altered mood patterns that are commonly seen in individuals with CFS. Research has repeatedly demonstrated that people with CFS are more likely to experience anxiety and depression. It is commonly known that mood problems and chronic illness are linked, but the relationship is especially significant when considering CFS. The constant exhaustion, the omnipresent doubt, the disturbance of the routine of life—all these things combine to cloud the soul.

The storey gets more intricate as we go deeper. The feeling of exhaustion is not just physical; it is also psychological. Feelings of hopelessness and powerlessness might result from the sense of being constantly exhausted, which exacerbates depression symptoms. In addition, the cognitive deficits that are frequently linked to CFS, like memory and focus issues, can exacerbate the emotional stress, resulting in a vicious cycle of misery and cognitive deterioration.

There are, nevertheless, refutations to take into account. Some others suggest that misdiagnosis or improper treatment of CFS may be the cause of the psychological symptoms, or perhaps the result. Critics could counter that the mental health problems are not a result of CFS but rather a core psychiatric condition. Is it possible that psychological anguish both precedes and increases the risk of developing CFS?

I address this with a refutation that is grounded in clinical practise and bolstered by an expanding corpus of research. Although mental health conditions can either precede or coexist with CFS, there appears to be a causal association between the two conditions based on the unique pattern of symptoms and the time interval between the start of CFS and psychological alterations. Before CFS manifests itself, many people report being in good mental health; psychological symptoms only appear as the illness worsens.

Furthermore, having a chronic illness that is frequently misdiagnosed can have a significant negative social and psychological impact. The psychological load of CFS is exacerbated by the loss of one's previous way of life, invalidation by those who do not comprehend the condition, and the fight to get proper treatment and recognition.

Research has demonstrated that treatments like graded exercise therapy (GET) and cognitive-behavioral therapy (CBT) can help manage CFS symptoms, including psychological distress, which is evidence of these psychological components. These results highlight the condition's intricacy and the interaction between the body and mind.

Think about this: How often do we undervalue the tenacity of people who struggle with mental illness in silence? And if we really paid attention to the stories of those who deal with CFS on a daily basis, could our understanding of the disorder change?

In summary, the psychological dimensions of chronic fatigue syndrome are not incidental elements within the broader narrative; rather, they play a pivotal role in moulding the experiences of those impacted by the disease. The path to wellness and the thorough management of CFS both depend on taking mental health issues into account. It is imperative, not optional, to address these psychological components in the holistic approach that I support.

So, as we close this chapter on our knowledge of CFS, let's write a new storey that recognises the richness of the human spirit and the nuanced interactions between the physical and psychological domains. By working together, utilising science, empathy, and the art of healing, we may shed light on the way to a deeper understanding of Chronic Fatigue Syndrome.

Daily Life With CFS

Daily Life with CFS

Picture waking up to a symphony of aches—the kind that clings to your body and won't go away even after your day's activities have come to an end. Jenna, a 42-year-old mother of two who works as a graphic designer and deals with the numerous difficulties caused by chronic fatigue syndrome (CFS) on a daily basis, follows this routine in the morning. Her narrative demonstrates ingenuity and tenacity in the face of an unseen foe.

Jenna's once-vibrant personal and professional lives were shrouded in a persistent veil of exhaustion. The main conflict she faced? A seemingly straightforward but unachievable goal is to have a "normal" day. The main problem with CFS is its debilitating tiredness, which is accompanied by a variety of symptoms that appear normal but are actually abnormal.

I entered Jenna's environment as a wellness advocate with the intention of changing her, not just treating her. We set out on a trip that called for a variety of tactics, each one specific to the rhythm of her life. Our strategy was all-encompassing, combining nutritional planning, psychological assistance, and other alternative therapies with lifestyle changes.

Our approach consisted of a series of thoughtful, small-scale steps rather than a miracle medication. We began with her nutrition, offering foods high in nutrients that would feed her body without overdoing it. In order to reduce stress and enhance the quality of sleep, we incorporated mild yoga and meditation. The psychological strategies that enabled Jenna to redraw the limits of her everyday activities and make sure that each one was a stride toward healing rather than a plunge into weariness were equally significant.

The outcome? Jenna started telling a different storey. She claimed to have more energy, have a clearer head, and be able to interact with her kids more completely. Her development was a slow dawn of vigour rather than an abrupt epiphany. The information, which included both her symptom diaries and sleep logs, reflected this upward trend and showed patterns that helped to clarify her hope.

Thinking back on Jenna's path gives us more comprehensive understanding. Although CFS can be a lonely struggle, it also serves as a wake-up call for a culture that is more understanding and caring. It emphasises the need for individualised care, proving that there is no one-size-fits-all approach to managing chronic illnesses.

Visual tools, like Jenna's energy and activity charts, help to crystallise her progress by providing concrete evidence of the invisible struggle that is being fought and progressively winning. Her charts are more than just lines and numbers; they are evidence of tenacity and the effectiveness of comprehensive intervention.

This storey runs throughout the broader picture of CFS management. It is a condition that necessitates a symphony of remedies, with each note representing the needs of the particular person. It shows us that mastering CFS is an act of harmony rather than conquest.

What about tomorrow, then? Could Jenna's tale serve as your guide on the CFS journey? Will the stillness of those who know the weight of exhaustion without words comfort you?

As we move on from Jenna's storey, consider this: What tiny adjustment can you make now that could have a big impact on your life with CFS?

Being a chronic fatigue syndrome sufferer involves more than just physical restrictions. It is also full with stories of adaptability and success, no matter how small. Every day is a painting, and although CFS may specify the colours, you are the one with the brush.

We've only just begun to explore the many facets of CFS management in this subchapter. As we continue, keep in mind that the key to conquering this illness is striking a careful balance between accepting its limitations and developing your inner power.

I'll leave you with this thought to ponder throughout the remainder of your day: what if the complexity of CFS is really a call to rediscover life's basic pleasures? Remember this question often as you work through the upcoming chapters. We will go deeper and reveal additional tactics and anecdotes in the pages that follow, giving you the knowledge and bravery to confront CFS with a healer's touch and a warrior's spirit.

Misconceptions and Myths

The people living in the sleepy hamlet of Serenityville, tucked away amid swaying willows and a placid lake, knew each other's pleasures and pains well. Here resided Maya, a lively high school instructor who was well-liked by both her pupils and other teachers. Her contagious laughter was a positive energy that frequently reverberated through the hallways.

But Maya's life took a sudden turn when she was always covered in a thick layer of exhaustion. Resting would not lift the curtain. The once-vivacious teacher had faded into obscurity. The problem was not only Maya's weariness; rather, it was the numerous myths surrounding her Chronic Fatigue Syndrome (CFS).

In my capacity as Maya's physician and health and wellness advisor, Dr. Ankita Kashyap, had to treat her illness while also debunking misconceptions that hindered her support network's comprehension. The trip was profoundly psychological and social in nature in addition to being medical.

It was a thorough approach. I put together a group of professionals who combined self-care, counselling, and nutrition specifically for Maya. We started a journey of lifestyle changes, using our bodies' and minds' combined abilities to help us through the confusing world of CFS.

The effects were subtle yet significant. Just like the first rays of dawn after a long night, Maya's strength started to return. She could return to her passion of teaching part-time. Despite being personal, this victory also demonstrated the effectiveness of holistic medicine.

When I thought back on Maya's case, I realised that the journey was about changing the perception of CFS rather than just treating symptoms. The lies that had previously prevented Maya from moving forward were now disintegrating, exposing the reality of her situation.

Take the widespread misconception that CFS is just "all in the mind," for example. We've heard that refrain how many times? Maya's narrative demonstrates that CFS is a multifaceted combination of biological, psychological, and environmental elements. It is a real thing, just as substantial as any medical issue, not a creation of the mind.

And what about the fallacy that fatigue alone is the only cause of CFS? Ah, if only things were that easy. A variety of symptoms, including post-exertional malaise—a condition in which even mild physical or mental exertion can cause an excessive and incapacitating drop in energy—are associated with the complex disease known as chronic fatigue syndrome.

Visual tools, such as the graph I used to monitor Maya's condition and development, gave us more than just information—they told a storey. It was a tale of highs and lows, tenacity and willpower. It was an effective weapon for demolishing falsehoods and putting understanding in their place.

Maya's experience serves as a microcosm for the larger field of CFS. It is a stark reminder to reconsider our strategy, to go over preconceptions and adopt a compassionate, fact-based narrative.

What lessons can you, the reader, take away from Maya's journey? Maybe it's the knowledge that CFS necessitates a complex viewpoint. Or perhaps it's the understanding that every CFS number hides a narrative, a person trying to maintain normalcy in the face of extreme exhaustion.

Are you prepared to challenge the misconceptions you've been taught about CFS? Are you willing to see the person behind the ailment and let empathy take the place of judgement?

Now let us go via the myth's lanes and reach the truth's boulevard. Let's begin with a straightforward but thought-provoking query: What if all you believed to be true about CFS was only the top of the iceberg?

Imagine all the Mayas in the world, no matter how many, struggling with this mysterious syndrome. Envision the resilience they gather daily to confront a world that frequently misinterprets their hardship.

It's time to dispel myths about CFS and expose its actual nature in order to bring light on the situation. This is about taking back lives, not just busting misconceptions.

Let's consider this as we wrap off this chapter: Are there any additional health and fitness misconceptions that we still cling to? How can society change to better assist persons who fight invisible conditions?

We will explore the realm of CFS in more detail in the pages that follow. We will examine the approaches, the healing, and the successes together. We shall discover that caring for someone with CFS is an art as well as a science, one that Maya and many others are gradually becoming experts in.

Greetings and welcome to "The Chronic Fatigue Syndrome Mastery Bible: Your Comprehensive Guide to Managing Chronic Fatigue Syndrome." Let's set out on a path of empowerment, healing, and discovery together.

Understanding Chronic Fatigue Syndrome

The History of CFS

The Enigmatic Tapestry of Chronic Fatigue Syndrome: A Historical Perspective

Have you ever considered how medical discoveries have come to be? How can they go from faint indications of symptoms to acknowledged ailments requiring medical attention and care? Such a road has been travelled by Chronic Fatigue Syndrome (CFS), a disorder that is as confusing as it is crippling. Its delicate weaving of science, culture, and the human experience becomes apparent as we untangle its fabric.

In the spirit of lively inquiry, let us take a trip back to the first days of CFS. Think back to the 1930s, when the polio outbreak was at its worst. Amid this crisis, a number of cases appeared that shared similar symptoms but were not polio. The severe exhaustion baffled doctors, but the term "myalgic encephalomyelitis" (ME) wasn't created until 1955 during an outbreak at the Royal Free Hospital in London. This was a crucial turning point in the development of what is today known as CFS.

However, why is this history relevant? Because knowing the CFS milestones influences how we address this complicated illness in the future and how we approach it in the present. Moving forward in time, the Lake Tahoe mystery illness was a major event of the 1980s. Here, CFS entered the American public consciousness and sparked a great deal of curiosity and investigation. Known as "Chronic Fatigue Syndrome" in 1988, this peculiar disease skirted the boundaries of scientific understanding, evading precise diagnosis like a shadow.

Diagrams that show symptom clusters and epidemiological spreading are examples of visual tools that help shed light on the mysterious nature of CFS. They provide witness to the medical community's tenacious search for solutions. Can you see the network of symptoms, each one serving as a clue that points to the central cause of CFS?

Regional and cultural differences have influenced how people view CFS over time. It is referred to as "Low Natural Killer Syndrome" in Japan, highlighting an important physiological discovery. In contrast, the British healthcare system struggled with ME, a diagnosis that is still prevalent in many Commonwealth countries. The complex, multidimensional nature of the disease itself is reflected in the multiplicity in nomenclature and interpretation.

As we approach the present, we observe that CFS is understood through contemporary interpretations and alterations. The 21st century has ushered in a period of genomics research, biotechnology, and a deeper exploration of the vast field of immunology. The 2015 Institute of Medicine (IOM) report, which aimed to improve and clarify the diagnostic procedure for CFS while highlighting its validity as a medical disorder, is one example of the emergence of new diagnostic criteria.

However, difficulties and disagreements accompany development. The realisation that CFS has a crippling effect on quality of life, similar to conditions like multiple sclerosis and chronic renal failure, marked a turning point in the discourse surrounding the illness. The dispute? a persistent lack of belief and stigma, with patients frequently written off as displaying psychosomatic symptoms—a charge that has dogged the CFS community for many years.

How can one look away from the passionate discussions around various treatment approaches, such as graded exercise therapy and cognitive-behavioral therapy? There are several disagreements in the CFS narrative regarding the effectiveness of immunomodulatory therapy, the significance of viral infections, and the mind-body relationship.

Let me question you now, reader: have you ever experienced a fatigue that persists even after resting? The disappointment of a disease that eludes a straightforward diagnosis? For people who have CFS, this is their daily existence. I, Dr. Ankita Kashyap, fervently support a holistic approach because this ailment calls for one. Together with my team, I advocate for a combination of dietary adjustments, customised nutrition plans, counselling, and complementary therapies. We value the power of community, alternative methods, and the dance of self-care in the management of CFS.

The narrative around CFS is never complete; it keeps changing with each new study, patient account, and clinical treatment. The illness that was once a whisper now demands our sympathies and our attention. It serves as a reminder that understanding is never a straight line but rather a complex tapestry of events and realisations.

In summary, chronic fatigue syndrome is a monument to the intricacy of human health and the tenacity of individuals who must traverse its seas. It is a disorder that has permeated every aspect of medical history and has developed in tandem with our comprehension of the human body and psyche. As we flip the page on CFS, we make room for the unwritten chapters that will go unwritten, the breakthroughs that will happen soon, and the hope that one day the mystery of CFS will be solved, providing comfort and answers to those who suffer from it.

As we continue to learn, treat, and advocate, let this historical perspective serve as both a reflection of the past and a beacon leading us toward compassionate care and comprehensive management of Chronic Fatigue Syndrome. Let's work together to forge a future in which CFS is not a death sentence, but rather a condition that is treated with understanding and a comprehensive, multifaceted approach to wellness.

Identifying Symptoms and Patterns

In the dark light of my clinic, I think back to the day that 34-year-old Maya, a graphic designer, entered the room; there, she exuded a weariness that words cannot express. She took with her her world, a disarray of unsolved issues and waning optimism, a microcosm of the daily struggles that many people with Chronic Fatigue Syndrome (CFS) face. Her path, like that of innumerable others, was marked by enigmatic symptoms that pretended to be nothing more than tiredness but were actually warning signs of a deeper illness.

Maya's difficulty was typical of the patients I treat. Her life, once full of energy and productivity, was now paralysed by excessive sluggishness, sleep deprivation, and a fog of thought that made even the most basic activities seem like monumental undertakings. Her experience serves as evidence of the widespread prevalence of CFS and the urgent need to solve its mysteries.

My approach to treating Maya's situation was holistic; it went beyond treating her physical health to include her mental, emotional, and even social aspects. We started making lifestyle changes, feeding her with a customised diet, and strengthening her mental health with psychological and counselling services. In order to restore her vitality, my team of experts and I created a tapestry of self-care practises, ranging from mild yoga to mindfulness activities.

Even though they happened gradually, the outcomes were profoundly altering. Maya's tiredness started to disappear like the tide going out, exposing the past version of herself. Clarity and fresh inventiveness replaced her cerebral fog, and the quality of her sleep increased. The graphic designer, who had previously doubted that she would come up with something brilliant, was now overflowing with ideas.

Thinking back on Maya's experience makes me think of the complex relationship that exists between CFS symptoms and patterns. While every patient's symptoms are different, they are all tied together with common threads, such as crippling exhaustion, trouble concentrating or remembering things, restless nights, sore muscles, and a host of other symptoms that come and go like the tides.

You may ask, though, why this matters to you. Imagine the power of realising that the whispers—or cries—that your own body makes could be the road map to taking back your life. That's exactly what we aim for when diagnosing and treating CFS symptoms.

Examine how these illnesses affect the common pleasures that many people take for granted as we analyse them. The shards of normalcy that CFS steals are the moments when one can wake up feeling rejuvenated, go for a stroll without worrying about burning out, or spend time doing something they love.

Let's envision this for a moment: Imagine an energy level graph, where each drop signifies a CFS patient's descent into exhaustion following seemingly insignificant activity. This would be a striking representation of the erratic character of the illness.

As we continue to put this jigsaw together, we need to question ourselves: What trends show up in these symptoms? How do they change in time with our everyday routines? Most importantly, though, is how we can use this information to empower people like Maya.

Imagine the possible cascading effects that could occur if patients were equipped with knowledge about their symptom patterns so they could prepare for and lessen the burden on their life. It's revolutionary—a retaking of power that CFS so frequently usurps.

But, there are hazards on this road. There are many arguments against the subjective character of CFS symptoms. The voices of the doubters are clear; they doubt the veracity of accounts such as Maya's. However, these critiques also contain the seeds of our commitment to learn more and give voice to the difficulties faced by persons with this syndrome.

By linking these unique accounts to the greater storey of CFS, we foster a sense of community empathy and a common goal of conquering this mysterious illness.

What might the appearance of your graph be? Are you able to chart the ups and downs of your energy, pinpointing the moments that send you reeling or the safe havens that provide you with a break?

This subchapter only scratches the surface of the complicated world of CFS, a disorder that is treatable despite its complexity. We get one step closer to taking back control of our lives with every symptom recognised and pattern recognised.

Let this thought remain with you as you turn the page: How could your life change if you could understand the language of your body's symptoms? The solution is found in the pages that follow, as we delve further into the tactics that have helped patients just like Maya find their way and can help you find yours as well.

Together, let's go out on this path to conquer chronic fatigue syndrome and recover not only our physical well-being but also our true essence of energy.

Diagnostic Criteria and Challenges

I met a woman whose tired eyes seemed to bear the weight of an invisible burden once, in the peaceful calm of my office, where the air is often pierced by the silent hope of recovery. Mother of two and graphic artist Sarah embodied the confounding conundrum that chronic fatigue syndrome (CFS) frequently presents. Like many others, she travelled a path filled with unresolved issues and a need for approval.

In the realm of CFS, Sarah faced a common challenge: a plethora of symptoms without a clear explanation, disregarded by some, and misinterpreted by many. The crux of her battle was figuring out a diagnosis that would account for her constant lethargy, mental fog, and a host of other illnesses that were linked to it.

For Sarah, as with many of my patients, there were several facets to the approach. We used a combination of diagnostic expertise and compassionate listening as we dug deeply into her medical history, way of life, and stressors. Since CFS is a syndrome for which there are no conclusive tests, it calls for close attention to detail and a broad perspective on health. We used the Centers for Disease Control and Prevention (CDC) criteria, which require the presence of a full range of symptoms, including pain, neurological problems, sleep abnormalities, and significant exhaustion that has persisted for more than six months.

Sarah had a complex treatment plan that included dietary changes, psychological support, and customised lifestyle modifications in addition to medicinal measures. We delved into the fields of light exercise regimens, cognitive behavioural therapy, and guided meditation, all of which strengthened her road to recovery.

Sarah did not experience immediate improvements, but she did experience significant ones. Gradually, the mist dissipated, and her vitality started to gradually rise. Her ability to resume part-time employment and spend more time with her kids was a direct result of her customised management plan's effectiveness.

In retrospect, Sarah's case highlighted the complex interactions that occur between a patient and a healthcare provider, the value of comprehensive treatment, and the significance of confirming a patient's experience. Although her path was not without difficulties, it demonstrated the possibility of resiliency and healing within the confines of CFS treatment.

Sarah's narrative serves as a witness to the difficulties and successes associated with identifying and treating CFS within the context of this work. It emphasises how important it is to have a caring, all-encompassing approach that recognises the complexity of the human situation.

Visual aids, including charts with symptom checklists and progress trackers, made Sarah's trip easier to see and gave her a concrete indicator of her success.

As the reader, would you not concur that the storey of CFS is more than just medical discourse? It's a human experience, and as such, it calls for a complex understanding braided with compassion and medical knowledge.

Now that we are moving from Sarah's tale to a more general conversation, we need to ask ourselves: how many other people walk this uncertain journey, and how can we, as a community of healers and fellow travellers, light the path ahead?

We so find ourselves at a juncture between reflection and action. For many people, chronic fatigue syndrome is a lived reality rather than just a collection of symptoms. What hope can we give to people who are still looking for answers, and how can we navigate this difficult terrain?

The Chronic Fatigue Syndrome Mastery Bible is more than simply a guidebook; it's a declaration of intent, an appeal to arms for people who want to comprehend and overcome this mysterious illness. Come along with me on this mastering adventure, as together we will solve the CFS puzzle and recover the vitality that is everyone's natural inheritance.

Psychological Impact of CFS

Imagine the predicament of 35-year-old graphic artist Sarah, whose life has been completely upended by Chronic Fatigue Syndrome, as the amber hues of morning begin to fade (CFS). Sarah, who was once a dynamic professional with a stellar reputation for her unwavering work ethic and inventive spark, now has a daily struggle with an unseen enemy that saps her vitality and leaves her exhausted all the time.

Sarah's primary obstacle is not just physical. One aspect of CFS that is often overlooked is the long-lasting shadow it creates across her mental and emotional landscape. We'll look at the tactics and fixes in this storey that Sarah used to get past her exhaustion and regain her strength of mind.

I was Sarah's physician, and I saw her first spiral into hopelessness. Her sense of reality was being eaten away by the unrelenting exhaustion, which was made worse by the doubts and incredulity of her colleagues and certain medical professionals. Our strategy started with validation, confirming that Sarah's experiences were real and worthy of consideration.

Our comprehensive approach integrated customised lifestyle adjustments, counselling, and a range of supplemental medicines. Sarah found it easier to express her frustrations and worries during regular sessions with a psychologist who specialised in chronic disease. She also gained methods to moderate her negative thought patterns using cognitive-behavioral strategies.

A crucial part was performed by nutrition. Sarah got the most energy-producing nutrients from her eating plan full of whole foods, and certain supplements addressed nutrient shortages that can worsen symptoms of chronic fatigue syndrome.

Despite it being strange, she included exercise in her routine. Her resilience was enhanced by gentle yoga and guided meditation, which strengthened her mind-body connection. This was about having a compassionate approach to movement, not about pushing past exhaustion.

The outcome? Sarah's experience had a profound impact. She continued to live with CFS, but within six months, she reported a 40% improvement in her energy levels. She was able to clear her head and resume her creative activities, albeit at a more deliberate pace.

When considering Sarah's situation in a broader context, it becomes evident that comprehensive care of CFS needs to give mental health just as much attention as it does physical symptoms. People who see these approaches as auxiliary rather than essential may criticise them, yet there is no denying the importance of the body and mind in healing.

Along the way, visual tools like Sarah's energy and mood diaries provided a strong source of motivation by showing the increasing trend in her well-being.

The main idea of this book—that mastering CFS necessitates a blueprint as unique as the person it serves—is connected to Sarah's life. It is about fostering a symbiotic relationship between the body and the mind, not just about treating symptoms.

What happens if you find yourself standing where Sarah used to be? What if your life's next chapter is one of empowerment and rejuvenation?

Imagine going to bed each day with the knowledge that you can rely on resources to provide you strength and comfort even in the midst of a storm. Turning the page and finding your own road to mastery is what "The Chronic Fatigue Syndrome Mastery Bible: Your Blueprint for Complete Chronic Fatigue Syndrome Management" promises.

The Science Behind CFS

I've seen the silent suffering of many people in the peaceful stillness of my clinic—a exhaustion so deep that it turns warriors into shadows of their former selves. Fatigue alone is not what Chronic Fatigue Syndrome (CFS) is all about; it is a relentless robber of energy. But what science is behind this mysterious illness? Let's take a tour through the complex web of data and hypotheses to try and solve the puzzle of CFS.

The claim that CFS is a complicated, multifaceted illness with a pathogenesis as elusive as a puff of smoke forms the basis of our investigation. It's the body's alarm system, warning that something is amiss in its fragile environment. The field of immunology provides our first light of knowledge. According to studies, CFS is largely caused by an immune system that is dysregulated. Pro-inflammatory cytokine levels are elevated in CFS patients, suggesting that their bodies are constantly on high alert, battling an invisible enemy.

As we dig farther, we find a landscape in which the regular ups and downs of energy production are disturbed. This disease has been linked to abnormalities in our cells' power plants, the mitochondria. Imagine a city where the electrical grid is failing; the energy wavers and wanes, bringing the once-bustling streets to a complete halt. For those with CFS, this is their everyday reality: their bodies struggle to produce the energy needed to complete even the most basic tasks.

However, we have to face refutations as we move over this terrain. Some argue that CFS is psychosomatic, a sign of mental illness as opposed to physical chaos. Although there is an undeniable biological connection between the mind and body, to dismiss CFS as only a psychological disorder would be to ignore the growing body of data. Research has shown that there is a physiological basis for the symptoms, as evidenced by the presence of neuroinflammation, which was identified by sophisticated imaging methods. The brain itself exhibits symptoms of distress.

The autonomic nerve system is another piece of the puzzle that appears beyond the immune system and energy generation. The disorder that affects our body's autonomic processes, known as dysautonomia, exerts its chaotic influence in CFS. Patients may experience unpredictability-related distress as a result of unconscious processes such as heart rate, blood pressure, and digestion that can get out of control.

The claim that CFS is a biological reality solidifies as we approach a resolution. Bit by piece, the data mounts up to paint a picture of a disease that is beyond easy explanation. Every body system contributes a discordant note to the symphony of malfunction. However, our comprehension is still far from perfect.

It is my desire that 'The Chronic Fatigue Syndrome Mastery Bible: Your Blueprint for Complete Chronic Fatigue Syndrome Management' acts as a beacon in this dance of light and dark, where science searches for solutions in the shadows. Because these pages provide not only science but also the means to rescue life from the grip of CFS. It is an empowerment trip that takes you from exhaustion to vigour and from comprehension to mastery.

I will thus leave you with this question: do we rise to the challenge of discovering an enigma's secrets or do we give up in the face of it? It is up to us, dear reader, to decide.

Debunking CFS Myths

Chronic fatigue syndrome, sometimes known as CFS, is a silent warrior that goes unnoticed by observers and occasionally even by people who experience it in the body's quiet battlegrounds. As I write this section of "The Chronic Fatigue Syndrome Mastery Bible: Your Blueprint for Complete Chronic Fatigue Syndrome Management," I am struck by how much the myths surrounding CFS have complicated the already difficult difficulties that my patients encounter.

Consider, if you will, a disorder shrouded in myth, where those who suffer from it are wrongfully accused of being indolent or of inflating their symptoms. For many people with CFS, this is their harsh reality. The sickness itself is not the only issue; the society narrative surrounding it is also problematic.

These fallacies have serious repercussions. People who have CFS are denied the emotional and medical help they require when it is not taken seriously. A mist of doubt obscures the way to recovery, leaving victims to fend for themselves—often alone—in it.

What if I told you, nevertheless, that we must begin piercing this cloud right now? Knowledge is our weapon, and effective communication is our tactic.

We must first illuminate the reality in order to debunk these falsehoods. CFS is a real illness with many facets that requires a customised approach to therapy. It is not a delusion. Our all-encompassing strategy includes dietary adjustments, customised nutrition, mental empowerment, and a range of complementary therapies that treat the full person.

Let's start by laying a foundation based on knowledge. We need to make it known to our patients, their families, and the general public that CFS is a legitimate medical disorder with precise diagnostic standards that calls for a careful, patient-centered approach to care.

The first step in putting this approach into practise is having talks in the media, in our communities, and in the clinic. Patients with CFS need our support, giving them a forum to talk about their experiences and get validation for their difficulties. By doing this, we upend the existing quo and promote a more sympathetic atmosphere.

However, don't just believe me; let's examine the supporting data. Research indicates that when individuals with CFS experience comprehension and encouragement, their ability to control their symptoms enhances. This is about observable gains in their physical well-being, not simply about feeling better emotionally.

Maybe you're wondering if there's anything else that can be done to dispel these beliefs. Undoubtedly, a multifaceted strategy is essential. It is imperative that appropriate instruction on CFS be provided to medical professionals during their training. Funding and public awareness of the condition's research are essential. All these paths hold great potential, but they all demand our steadfast dedication.

Imagine a society in which CFS is viewed as an issue that is handled with knowledge and compassion rather than as a diagnosis that is murmured and laced with judgement. This is the future we can build and the one we aim for.

Now, you might be wondering, "What can I do?" The solution is straightforward yet effective: learn for yourself, impart what you know, and help people around you. Every discussion that dispels a myth and every piece that clarifies the conditions around CFS is a step in the right direction toward that better future.

Never undervalue the influence of personal narratives. We highlight the intricacy of CFS and the courage required to deal with it on a daily basis by sharing the experiences of those who live with it.

These stories have the ability to touch people's emotions, humanise them, and influence their opinions.

To sum up, never forget that compassion grows with understanding. We are cultivating a garden of support and affirmation for individuals impacted by Chronic Fatigue Syndrome while we strive to dispel the myths surrounding it. Together, we can gradually change the perception of CFS by eroding isolation and stigma and substituting understanding and support.

This chapter is merely one thread in the larger fabric we weave, a fabric that depicts resiliency, fought battles, and future triumphs. Come along with me, Dr. Ankita Kashyap, as we debunk the misconceptions and expose the facts in "The Chronic Fatigue Syndrome Mastery Bible" and go on a path to conquer CFS.

Patient Stories: The Human Perspective

Mother of two Sarah, 35, was a graphic designer confronting an unending dawn of her own in the peaceful suburb of Westville, where the morning air is crisp with the promise of the day. In the rush of everyday activity, she was shrouded in an unexplainable weariness that dampened her formerly lively lifestyle.

Sarah's journey into Chronic Fatigue Syndrome (CFS) started with mild symptoms that developed into a debilitating daily battle. Her eyes, which were a monument to the human spirit's tenacity, screamed volumes about the quiet struggles she had faced as I sat across from her.

Sarah's biggest struggle was a chronic state of exhaustion that kept her confined to her bed and made her days seem like a haze of moments only partially experienced. This was not the kind of lethargy that could be remedied by getting a good night's sleep.

We decided to take a multifaceted approach, mirroring the intricacy of CFS with our customised method. We went over her food, her lifestyle, and her mental health, making adjustments to each that would help her feel better. Self-help strategies gave her the ability to chip away at the psychological stones dragging her down, while counselling sessions revealed which ones they were.

Small victories—moments when Sarah freed portions of her life from the grip of exhaustion—interspersed Sarah's journey. We strengthened her body with the nutrients it had been longing for by introducing foods through careful diet planning that ended up becoming allies in her battle.

Alternative forms of treatment also had an impact. Her energy levels increased as a result of the combination of the healing scents of aromatherapy, the meditative flow of yoga, and the soft touch of acupuncture needles. Every modality was a note in the beautiful melody of recovery, creating a symphony of wellness.

The outcome? Evidence of the effectiveness of a comprehensive strategy. After being exhausted, Sarah's energy started to surge like the rising tide. Data gathered over several months revealed an improving trend, with each day seeming slightly brighter and livelier. Despite their usefulness, the graphs and charts were unable to depict the vitality and vibrancy of her laughter, or the spark that was once again in her eyes or cheeks.

When one considers Sarah's narrative, it becomes evident that mental health is just as important as physical health in the fight against CFS. Two people dance together, with each step requiring a careful balancing act between mental and physical health. Sarah's narrative is just one example, a solitary strand in the vast fabric of human perseverance.

How can one not stop to think about the significant consequences of a trip like this? What does it indicate about the way we see health and the unseen struggles that countless people face?

Allow Sarah's narrative to serve as a lighthouse and a guide for you as you turn the pages of this book and navigate the murky waters of CFS. Her storey is entwined with the more general ideas of holistic health, serving as a reminder that every patient is an individual universe in need of a customised road map to navigate their distinct constellation of symptoms.

What does it mean to hear a patient's narrative all the way through? To hear the words unsaid, to comprehend the silent cry for assistance? Every healthcare professional should ponder this topic; it is a quiet voice that directs our hands and hearts.

Now let's move from the individual to the group, from the particular to the general. Keep in mind the people behind the numbers and the narratives behind the facts as we delve deeper into the nuances of CFS. Because the real key to beating Chronic Fatigue Syndrome lies in the stories of people just like Sarah.

And so, my dear reader, I leave you with this question: Is it possible to truly grasp a condition as complicated as CFS without accepting the human perspective and without comprehending the patient narratives that form the core of our entire journey toward well-being?

Every success storey serves as a lighthouse, pointing the way toward a more humane and efficient method of healing. These narratives serve as the basis for the comprehensive care of Chronic Fatigue Syndrome, a dynamic blueprint that changes constantly in tandem with the lives it aims to improve.

Diagnostic Pathways

Recognizing the Signs

The subtlety of Chronic Fatigue Syndrome (CFS) frequently whispers before it screams in the maze of symptoms that the human body might exhibit. For many who are lost on the unpredictable route of this ailment, early discovery can be their guiding light. Together, let's clear this road and discover how to spot CFS's early warning signals.

Envision, if you will, the start of a typical workday in a busy city. Emma, a graphic artist whose life is a colourful tapestry of deadlines and dreams, is introduced to us at this point. However, the threads have been fraying recently. She has been experiencing a chronic tiredness that seems to be unaffected by sleep. Emma's tale is a case study in the intricacy of CFS onset, not just about fatigue.

The primary obstacle manifested as a sneaky thief of energy. Emma, who was always lively and unflappable, started to exhibit an unexplained fatigue. It was a profound lethargy that clung to her bones like ivy, not the kind that comes after a hard day's work or a restless night.

The solution to her dilemma was multidimensional. Together, my team and I used our combined knowledge to create a customised plan that included nutritional changes, stress reduction methods, and a moderate but regular exercise schedule. Our goal was to provide Emma with self-help tools and knowledge that she could easily incorporate into her everyday routine.

Though they took time to manifest, the effects were significant. Week by week, Emma started to feel more alive. Her slumber grew more rejuvenating, and the thick veil of exhaustion parted, exposing her once again as the vibrant professional that she was. Emma's increased performance at work and her restored participation in social activities were concrete indicators of her rehabilitation, thus these results went beyond being just subjective.

When one considers Emma's journey, it is evident how important early detection and intervention are. Although the tactics we used weren't novel in and of themselves, their specific application made them revolutionary. Every CFS case is different and needs a custom solution.

While graphs may not be appropriate for this storey, consider one that shows Emma's energy levels over time. As each tactic takes root, the original flatline starts to curve and gradually rises upward, providing a visual record of her development.

Emma's experience highlights the value of a customised approach, which links it to the greater topic of CFS management. Since no two circumstances are the same, our best resources are adaptability and attentiveness.

What if Emma had disregarded those first murmurs? Could she have carried on with her career and lived her life with the same fervour she was used to? This question nags at us, making us think about the terrible effects of ignoring symptoms.

The intricacies of CFS can go unnoticed because they mimic normal wear and tear. Telltale indicators, though, can help distinguish the early stages of this illness from fatigue that is just normal. Have you ever experienced extreme weariness that was unabated by sleep? Have you ever had a mental fog, feeling as if a web has entangled your thoughts?

It's important to pay close attention to your body. A deeper malaise can be indicated by a chronic sore throat, inexplicable muscle soreness, new or severe headaches, and great weariness following physical or mental exertion. Early diagnosis and recognition of these symptoms are essential, as awareness is the first step towards conquering CFS.

It is important to keep in mind that dealing with CFS is a marathon rather than a sprint. It takes time, persistence, and—above all—courage to ask for assistance as soon as you see the first symptoms. It is crucial to embrace a wide range of treatment approaches, from self-care and psychological support to exercise and diet.

Let's consider the significance of identifying these indications as we wrap up this chapter. Early identification slows the syndrome's course and opens the door to more efficient treatment. It's the first move in regaining control and igniting the vigour that CFS is trying to put out.

Emma's narrative serves as a ray of hope and an example of the value of prompt diagnosis and customised treatment. Remember that when we go through "The Chronic Fatigue Syndrome Mastery Bible," it is not just medical experts who can master this condition—awareness everyone's and actions matter as well.

Let us move forward, believing that life can be enjoyed to the fullest, that CFS can be controlled, and that vitality can be restored with every new page turned. Recall that you have the ability to alter the course of your own storey if you pay close attention to the whispers of CFS. They don't have to become shouts.

Consulting With Healthcare Providers

Picture yourself slogging through a fog, an engulfing mist that follows you everywhere you go. It's Chronic Fatigue Syndrome (CFS), an intriguing condition that casts a shadow over your life rather than the romantic mist that poets long for. Your trusted healthcare providers are your map and compass on your journey. But how can you make your way through the confusing landscape of medical advice and interventions? Let me lead the way for you.

The first step on the path is acknowledging a sobering fact: diagnosing CFS is notoriously challenging. A confusing diagnostic maze that can leave you feeling confused is created by symptoms that overlap with a multitude of other ailments. The difficulty? to locate a medical professional that views you as an individual on a journey toward wellness rather than just as a collection of symptoms.

If neglected, the result is a downward spiral of annoyance and lost chances for assistance. Imagine the horror of receiving therapies that, because they are directed at the incorrect opponent, do not relieve your exhaustion. A life spent chasing shadows rather than welcoming the light of appropriate care carries a significant risk.

Creating a collaboration with medical professionals who are not just expert practitioners but also empathetic hearers is the answer. It is your task to locate allies who are prepared to fight CFS with a combination of empathy and rigour in the trenches alongside you.

Before beginning this mission, preparation is necessary. This is how you will fight:

1. : Enter the consultation room equipped with a detailed symptom diary. This log is more than simply a journal; it's a storey of your life with CFS that illustrates the ups and downs of your energy waves.

2. : When communicating with doctors, clarity is key. Explain your experiences in a way that medical practitioners can understand.

For example, "unrelenting exhaustion that impedes daily activities" is what fatigue turns into.

3. : Assert your needs with the confidence of someone who knows their own body. Keep in mind that you are the authority on your symptoms.

4. : Look for providers with a track record of treating CFS or related disorders. These are the knowledgeable guides you require.

5.: Take into account interdisciplinary teams that combine traditional and complementary medicine, mirroring my own all-encompassing therapeutic strategy.

I've seen firsthand how effective this tactic can be. Patients who previously felt invisible have gained a voice and access to therapies that actually improve their condition. It's not just anecdotal, research indicates that collaborations between patients and doctors can result in more precise diagnosis and efficient treatment regimens.

Obviously, there are other options. In support groups, where members share their tales and act as a collective compass, some patients find comfort. Some people rely on internet resources, searching through the vast digital space for direction. Although these resources provide assistance, the knowledge of healthcare professionals should be complemented rather than replaced.

The management of chronic fatigue syndrome is a multifaceted approach that involves perseverance, tolerance, and collaboration. With "The Chronic Fatigue Syndrome Mastery Bible," as you turn the pages of your journey, keep in mind that the correct healthcare provider is a co-author of your storey of recovery as well as a consultant. You may write a narrative of healing and optimism together.

Diagnostic Criteria for CFS

Imagine losing energy before you even get out of bed every day because you feel like an invisible weight is bearing down on your chest when you wake up. Imagine attempting to explain this unseen battle to people who inquire only to encounter cynicism. For many people suffering from Chronic Fatigue Syndrome (CFS), which is frequently misdiagnosed and misunderstood, this is their reality. But how do doctors determine a diagnosis for a disease that is so mysterious and pervasive?

Starting the process of diagnosing CFS is like trying to find your way through a maze; you need to be patient, pay close attention to details, and realise that not everyone who wanders is lost. The key to making the diagnosis is to discover a group of clinical manifestations that meet the predetermined criteria, rather than focusing on a single pathognomonic symptom or test.

The primary component of a CFS diagnosis is, first and foremost, a persistent or relapsing fatigue with a new or distinct onset, not related to continuous exertion, not significantly alleviated by rest, and leading to a marked reduction in prior levels of social, educational, occupational, or personal activities. Patients describe this intense exhaustion as literally changing their lives—the kind that creeps into the very marrow of your bones. Have you ever been so exhausted that even the most straightforward chore seems impossible?

Medical professionals seek for concomitant symptoms that have lasted for at least six months in addition to this extreme weariness. Post-exertional malaise, or a worsening of symptoms after physical or mental exertion that would not have elicited such a reaction prior to the disease, is one of these symptoms, but it is not the only one. Imagine your ordinary routine turning into an impossible task, like climbing a single flight of stairs to become your Everest.

Even worse, a lot of patients complain about their sleep being unrefreshing—a terrible irony for those who spend their nights trying to get some shut-eye. They suffer from significant short-term memory loss or concentration problems, commonly known as "brain fog," in which ideas appear to elude them like water between fingers.

But the symptoms of CFS are a far more complex tapestry. Fatigue is typically accompanied by a plethora of other illnesses, including headaches of a different kind or intensity, painful lymph nodes, muscle discomfort, multi-joint pain without redness or swelling, and recurrent or persistent sore throats. These symptoms are the knots that make it challenging to understand the underlying cause of the patient's distress, not just strands in the cloth of their existence.

In addition to ruling out other potential medical and mental disorders that could account for the symptoms, doctors must diagnose CFS. Differential diagnosis calls for a thorough assessment that includes a thorough medical history, a physical examination, a mental health assessment, and specific laboratory testing. However, what about the disorders that are concealed and seem as CFS? It is necessary to take into account and rule out conditions including autoimmune illnesses, sleep difficulties, mental health conditions, and hypothyroidism.

It is clear that diagnosing CFS is difficult. It is a diagnostic of inclusion rather than exclusion, in which a particular tune is sung by a harmonic chorus of symptoms. It is the medical professional's responsibility to pay close attention to this melody, dissect the harmonics, and determine the CFS tune.

In my capacity as a health and wellness professional who values a holistic approach, I implore my clients and other medical professionals to pay close attention to the stories of people who are impacted by CFS. Because their tales include hints that, when deciphered with clinical dexterity, can result in a diagnosis and, eventually, a course toward treatment.

It is impossible to overestimate the significance of dietary planning, counselling, lifestyle changes, and psychological support in the management of CFS. These interventions serve as the cornerstone upon which a patient's quality of life can be gradually restored, day by day, brick by brick.

CFS is a feeling, experienced, and lived illness rather than one that may be detected by a blood test or X-ray. It necessitates a thorough, sympathetic approach to diagnosis and treatment that takes into account the needs of the body, mind, and soul.

To sum up, the CFS diagnostic criteria are an essential road map for traversing the challenging terrain of this illness. They serve as a compass that points both patients and medical professionals in the direction of comprehension, acceptance, and hope. Let us keep in mind that the first step toward mastery is acknowledging the beginning of the journey as we flip the pages of this Chronic Fatigue Syndrome Mastery Bible. For those impacted by CFS, comprehending the diagnostic criteria is the first step toward empowerment and wellbeing.

So, dear reader, let me leave you with this thought: How can we all step in unison with compassion and knowledge to support those who suffer from Chronic Fatigue Syndrome during the complex dance of diagnosis and treatment? As we continue to examine the broad field of CFS management, let's consider this.

Tests and Assessments

Unraveling the Enigma of Chronic Fatigue Syndrome

Have you ever experienced the weight of tiredness enveloping you, making even the most mundane activities feel like impossible undertakings? Envision that sensation continuing for months on end, unrelenting and inexplicable. This is the world of an individual suffering from Chronic Fatigue Syndrome (CFS), an intricate ailment that has baffled the medical profession for many years. Now that we have covered this important subchapter, let's explore the maze of exams and evaluations that are essential markers on the way to comprehending and treating CFS.

The basic claim of our search is that a comprehensive approach is necessary for an accurate diagnosis of CFS, which is a complex process that involves more than just tests. In order to piece together this illness, a number of tests are used, not so much to confirm CFS (there isn't a single test for that), but rather to rule out other illnesses that could be masquerading as CFS.

The Centers for Disease Control and Prevention and other medical organisations' suggested practises serve as the main source of proof for this claim (CDC). They recommend a comprehensive assessment that consists of a physical examination, a full history, and a well-chosen set of laboratory testing. But shall we take a closer look at this?

Envision a patient, Maya, who arrives at my clinic covered in the exhaustion of unidentified persistent fatigue. An extensive blood panel is required as the initial step. This is not a hunt for CFS markers because none have been found yet; rather, it is a search for imposters, such as vitamin deficiencies, thyroid issues, or anaemia, which can resemble symptoms of CFS.

We investigate further, delving into Maya's intricate bodily functions. Tests including immune system panels, inflammatory markers, and hormonal assays help us comprehend her disease by removing a layer at a time. However, because of the intricacy of CFS, normal test findings are frequently the rule rather than the exception. Here, as we decipher the silences between the notes of her test findings, science and the art of medicine dance together.

Here's the twist, though: There is evidence to contradict the claims made by some individuals with normal test results, who are quickly diagnosed with CFS and told their symptoms are psychosomatic. We have to refute this storyline. As an advocate of complementary and alternative medicine, I firmly believe that CFS is a real biological illness, and that a patient's sense of sickness is not invalidated by the lack of aberrant test results.

In support of this, I offer the use of specialist tests such as the tilt table test, which evaluates the body's response to positional changes and may reveal dysautonomia, a common co-occurring condition with CFS. Furthermore, exercise tolerance tests may detect the post-exertional malaise that is a defining feature of chronic fatigue syndrome (CFS), and sleep investigations may uncover disturbances that are invisible to the tired eye.

However, the adventure doesn't finish with exams. The patient narratives, their symptom patterns, and how these affect their day-to-day lives are all equally important. It involves making the connections between seemingly unrelated symptoms and creating a clear picture of their overall health.

Let us now turn our attention to a conclusion that supports our first claim. The diagnosis of CFS is a complex mosaic made from clinical expertise, a range of examinations, and a sympathetic comprehension of the patient's reality. By using this comprehensive strategy, we provide ourselves with the knowledge necessary to direct our patients toward wellness and negotiate the murky seas of CFS.

I want to leave you with a thought as we wrap up this subchapter: Given how difficult it is to diagnose CFS, how resilient are people who deal with illness on a daily basis? Let their fortitude serve as evidence of the seriousness of their illness and our dedication to providing for it. We shall go deeper into the subtleties of Chronic Fatigue Syndrome in the pages that follow, but for now, let's take a moment to recognise the bravery needed to persevere and the diligence needed to comprehend.

Challenges in CFS Diagnosis

Imagine a disease that is so mysterious that its very name causes controversy, where the symptoms are inconsistent with a wide range of other ailments and defy precise diagnosis standards. This is the world of chronic fatigue syndrome (CFS), which I, Dr. Ankita Kashyap, walk with my patients through on a daily basis. To help them understand the complexities of this illness, I use an integrated and holistic approach.

Maria, a thirty-five-year-old graphic designer, walks into my clinic as dawn breaks over the quiet town. Her eyes, which were once bright, now seem heavy with unexplained fatigue. Many others in similar situations can relate to her experience of overcoming numerous medical offices, which serves as a testament to her tenacity.

The Obstacle: Maria's chronic weariness, which is not relieved by rest and is accompanied by musculoskeletal pain, cognitive decline, and other symptoms, has become her shadow. She embodies the main difficulties in diagnosing CFS, including the lack of a conclusive test, symptoms that can be confused with other illnesses, and the scepticism she encounters.

Approach: In my work, we go in-depth. We eliminate the typical suspects, such as depression, anaemia, and thyroid issues. We investigate less-traveled territory, looking for immunological deficiencies, hormonal abnormalities, and viral triggers. Gaining clarity is a step closer with each stone turned.

Maria had a difficult voyage. Test results are not definitive. Still, we don't give up. We work with a multidisciplinary team that includes alternative health practitioners, psychologists, and nutritionists. A customised, high-nutrient eating plan is created to reduce inflammation and increase vitality. Her relationship with weariness is intended to be reframed during cognitive-behavioral therapy sessions, and mindfulness meditation cultivates a sense of control.

Results: Maria's vitality gradually but noticeably blossoms over months. Her energy levels have increased by thirty percent, her discomfort has subsided, and her fog has cleared in her mind. Although there is little data in this area, each patient's advancement strengthens our belief.

Thought: The path with CFS is a patchwork of mistakes made along the way. Maria's situation illustrates the perseverance needed on the part of patients as well as professionals. There are several criticisms, including the psychological toll on patients, peer scepticism, and the absence of widely acknowledged standards. Still, progress is forged by these fires.

Visual Supports: My office walls are covered in charts that show the progression of therapy, dietary modifications, and symptom patterns—all vital tools in our toolbox against the elusiveness of CFS.

Linking Up with the Main Story: Maria's storey is only one part of the CFS puzzle. The narrative of each sufferer is interwoven with the larger problem of comprehending and treating this disease. Our all-encompassing approach aims to empower individuals to take back control of their life rather than only treat their symptoms.

Transitional Thought: However, what about individuals who are still lost in the maze of unidentified persistent exhaustion? How many Marias are there who are waiting to have their struggles acknowledged?

Let us consider the silent struggles, the invisible triumphs, and the unwavering human spirit that endures despite exhaustion as we flip the pages of this Mastery Bible. One patient at a time, one breakthrough at a time, we are collectively getting closer to conquering Chronic Fatigue Syndrome.

And now, dear reader, as you take in the core of Maria's journey and the complex issues it raises, I ask you to consider how society as a whole might be able to better support people who are struggling with the mystery of CFS. In the face of such a confusing enemy, how can we cultivate an atmosphere of empathy, comprehension, and unwavering research?

Although the path to mastery is arduous, we get stronger, wiser, and better prepared to meet the obstacles that lie ahead with every step we take. Come along with me as we explore the depths of Chronic Fatigue Syndrome and come out on the other side with a comprehensive management blueprint that is a monument to the human spirit's resiliency and the efficacy of integrated, patient-centered care.

Second Opinions and Specialist Referrals

Getting Through the Complicated Maze of Chronic Fatigue Syndrome: The Value of Specialist Referrals and Second Opinions

Have you ever been at the intersection of hope and doubt, wishing there was a clear solution to your ongoing fatigue? These points are all too prevalent in the confusing search to comprehend Chronic Fatigue Syndrome (CFS). This is where things get really important: deciding whether to get a second view or professional advice.

The path of having CFS is paved with uncertainty. A diagnosis might be difficult to come by, and the relief-bringing treatments are frequently as individual as the people who need them. This is the dilemma we deal with in the field of managing CFS; it's the main obstacle that can make or break our journey toward recovery.

Consider, for example, a situation in which this crucial phase is skipped. For a patient, what does it mean? Misdiagnosis, mishandling, or maybe failing to recognise an underlying illness that presents as CFS. The repercussions could be disastrous: a recurrence of symptoms, possible health decline, and a subtle eroding of hope.

A glimmer of hope amidst this intricacy is the judicious seeking of second views and specialised recommendations. This is a calculated move to address a complex ailment, not a betrayal of confidence in one's primary care physician. It's a step that represents advocating for one's health and empowerment.

So how does this actually get put into practise? The procedure is simple, but it requires attention to detail. Start by explaining to your present healthcare provider your worries and the reasons behind your need for additional information. Ask to be referred to professionals who specialise in CFS or the symptoms you are facing.

This approach has a wealth of anecdotal evidence backing it up, as well as innumerable accounts from patients who resolved their problems and found comfort in changing their viewpoint. It is seen in the comfort that follows from a more individualised treatment programme that takes into account the various symptom combinations that each patient may encounter.

But what if we don't find the answers we're looking for along this path? This is where it's important to keep in mind that there are a plethora of options to consider when managing CFS. Novel medicines, ongoing research, and integrative techniques are all promising avenues for alternate answers.

In this storey, every line develops like a petal in a flower of comprehension. It is evident from the imagery that managing CFS is an organic process that calls for tender care rather than a straight line. Is it possible that by consulting another person, we are creating a whole new world for ourselves?

Every time a specialist visits, more knowledge is added. We act like archaeologists, carefully removing the layers of doubt to uncover the remnants of our health below. This procedure is not only advantageous but also necessary. It serves as our compass in navigating the mist of chronic illness.

Now think about how this journey's rhythms—the tempo of visits, the symphony of expert opinions—all work together to produce a concerto of all-encompassing care. There is a heart to this rhythm that speaks to healing.

Remembering the strength of the patient's voice in this tune is important. Your personal narrative, life lessons learned, and observations are what drive the fight against CFS. Patient-physician communication is transformational rather than merely transactional.

As we come to an end, consider the importance of what you have just been presented with. Accept the idea that getting second opinions and specialist referrals is a path to potential in the management of CFS, not a side trip. It is evidence of the tenacity and willpower that characterise the human spirit.

Let's move seamlessly into the next section of our conversation with the knowledge that, despite CFS being a formidable foe, we can handle it by employing tact and intelligence. We are getting closer to mastery with every step we take—mastery over our own fate in the field of health and wellness, not just over a condition.

Accepting the Diagnosis

There are those among us for whom the warm glimmer of dawn signals a different kind of reality, one in which getting out of bed can seem like an impossible effort. These people experience reality differently than the rest of us. This is the life of someone living with Chronic Fatigue Syndrome (CFS), a disorder that has been misunderstood and hidden for far too long.

It can be as confusing as it is relieving to receive a diagnosis that sets the course for living with CFS. It can provide some relief to finally have a name for the illness after months or even years of inexplicable symptoms. The acceptance of a diagnosis that is both validating and life-altering, however, is where a big problem occurs.

It can be difficult to embrace Chronic Fatigue Syndrome as a legitimate and important aspect of one's life. The mind resists; accepting an illness that necessitates significant lifestyle adjustments and offers no short cures is difficult. This is where things get tricky: refusing to accept the diagnosis can make CFS worse, which can set off a crippling cycle of stress, deteriorating symptoms, and hopelessness.

What occurs if the challenge is not met? The effects may cascade, impacting not just an individual's well-being but also their interpersonal connections, career goals, and general standard of living. One cannot stress how urgent it is to solve this issue.

Nevertheless, there is a way out of this maze of ambiguity, one that I, Dr. Ankita Kashyap, have developed over many years of clinical and research experience. This strategy focuses on forming a partnership with the adversity and using it as a catalyst for transformation, rather than ignoring it.

Recognition is the first step towards a solution. Recognize that you have CFS and allow yourself to experience all of the associated feelings, such as grief, rage, and frustration. This is the first step to taking back control of your life, not a sign of surrender.

Next, get knowledgeable. In the darkness of ignorance, knowledge shines like a beacon, empowering those who possess it. Find out more about CFS, its effects, and its symptoms. You start to tame the beast by comprehending it.

The next step is to put together your support system, which should consist of loved ones, CFS warriors, and medical experts. Even if you are the ship's captain, a crew is still necessary.

Once your team is in place, create a management strategy that suits your particular requirements. This approach should include dietary adjustments, alternative therapies, psychological assistance, and a balanced lifestyle. It's more about a patchwork of interventions sewn together to enhance your well-being than it is about a single, universal cure.

I have seen amazing gains in my work when these strategies are put into practise. Patients report feeling more energised and hopeful after feeling lost in a sea of exhaustion. They describe a life that is informed by CFS rather than defined by it, one in which every tiny accomplishment is cherished.

There are, of course, other options, such concentrating only on medical care or challenging one's body's limitations in spite of the diagnosis. However, these routes frequently result in advantages that are fleeting at the expense of long-term wellbeing. Although the integrated strategy I support is not the simple one, it is one that leads to long-term benefits.

Imagine living a life in which you are in charge and CFS does not rule every decision you make. Imagine waking up to mornings that are full of opportunities rather than constraints. This isn't just a far-off fantasy—acceptance is the key that opens the door and makes it a possible reality.

Now ask yourself if you're prepared to start this adventure with a step. Can you accept the diagnosis as a fresh start rather than a death sentence?

This acceptance is an active decision rather than a passive one. Every decision you make gives you the opportunity to change the course of your life and live not in the darkness of chronic fatigue syndrome but rather in the light of your own resilience.

As you choose this route, keep in mind that accepting oneself is a team effort. Make a connection, reach out, and use the cumulative experience of those who have travelled this path to direct you. By working together, we can overcome the difficulties caused by CFS and use them as stepping stones to a full and active life.

The most important realisation regarding chronic fatigue syndrome is that, although it is a component of your life, it is not the weaver. Indeed, you are. You weave a life lived with intention, grace, and an unwavering spirit—a masterpiece of your own design—with every strand of acceptance, knowledge, support, and self-care.

Recognizing your diagnosis is only the beginning of a canvas waiting to be painted with your distinct hues. Let's depict a future free from Chronic Fatigue Syndrome marked by resiliency, hope, and mastery. Together, we will compose a wellness symphony that touches the core of who we are and reverberates throughout the lives of those who require its melodies.

As this chapter comes to an end, I hope you are inspired to turn the page and intrigued to learn about the comprehensive Chronic Fatigue Syndrome management guide that is within of you. This is a glorious beginning, not the end.

Medical Management of CFS

First Steps After Diagnosis

Today marks the start of a new chapter. You could experience a range of feelings after receiving a diagnosis of Chronic Fatigue Syndrome (CFS), including relief, perplexity, and concern. However, keep in mind that you are not alone during the storm. You will receive kind and resilient guidance from me, Dr. Ankita Kashyap, as you navigate the complex world of managing this illness. As we go out on this road, let's keep one thing in mind: building a strong foundation for efficient CFS management.

You need to assemble your toolkit before we go into the specifics of this roadmap: a healthcare team that is supportive, a notebook that you can use to track your symptoms and progress, and an open mind that is willing to adapt. You can start with these conditions met.

Picture a map with every route representing a step toward improved health. Our comprehensive package comprises initial consultations, lifestyle evaluations, and the development of an individualised treatment plan. They work together to create the framework for your management approach.

Now, let's navigate each step with care.

The first step is a thorough medical assessment. Make follow-up meetings with your primary care physician and think about speaking with a CFS expert after receiving your diagnosis. They will assist in validating your diagnosis and helping to rule out any other ailments. Have you scheduled these meetings yet? Otherwise, put them in your planner right now.

We then need to evaluate your way of life as it is. Examining your food, exercise regimen, sleep habits, and stress levels are all part of this. Do they help or hurt your overall wellbeing? Record your observations in a journal. When you meet with your healthcare team to talk about modifications, it will be a useful tool.

Step three is creating your customised care plan. This is your manifesto for life with CFS, not just any old document. It will cover food suggestions, low-impact workout routines, and energy-pacing techniques. I, along with your healthcare team, will assist you in developing a plan that is both practical and long-lasting.

I invite you to adopt the following slogan as we delve deeper: "Small adjustments, huge impact." Start with a sleep regimen that restores your body and a diet that gradually incorporates foods high in nutrients. Do you sense the seeds of change beginning to sprout?

But exercise caution—overdoing it is a common mistake. It's important to pace. Recall that the journey towards healing is a journey, not a sprint. Pay attention to your body and honour its limitations.

How do you tell if you're headed in the correct direction? There will be more "good days" than terrible ones, you'll notice. Even modest improvements, like an increase in energy or a better night's sleep, will show up in your notebook as a trend of consistent progress. Appreciate these successes since they show that your body is reacting to your hard work.

If you experience obstacles, don't give up. There may be flare-ups, so it's critical to review your treatment plan with your team and make the required modifications. This is an opportunity to refine your approach, not a sign of failure.

Let's take a brief break. Consider the data that was presented. Could you see yourself doing these actions? Is the route you are on beginning to take shape? You are the guide on this revolutionary adventure that is just getting started.

Finally, dear reader, keep in mind that although the initial steps following a CFS diagnosis may feel overwhelming, you can confidently manage your disease if you have a well-defined plan and a team that supports you. Maintain a close notebook, an open mind, and a mentality that is open to accepting change. One step at a time, we shall walk this journey together.

This subsection only provides a brief overview of "The Chronic Fatigue Syndrome Mastery Bible." Each page will provide you with information, tactics, and hope as we go along. Here is your guide to managing Chronic Fatigue Syndrome from start to finish. Greetings from a life where you are in control of your health.

Pharmacological Interventions

- Navigating the Medicinal Maze

Envision, if you will, a maze-like garden where every path leads to relief, yet the right turn is never easy to find. This is the path that many people with Chronic Fatigue Syndrome (CFS), a complicated illness that is difficult to treat and frequently misdiagnosed, take. As Dr. Ankita Kashyap, I have seen innumerable patients struggle and succeed. Today, I want to share with you a case that highlights the complexities of pharmaceutical treatments in the treatment of chronic fatigue syndrome.

Aarav was a 38-year-old software engineer whose life was cut short by the crippling hold of CFS. He resided in the bustling city of New Delhi. Aarav was once a dynamic professional, but his constant exhaustion, cognitive impairments, and muscle aches reduced him to a shell of his former self.

The lack of a universally effective treatment for CFS posed the biggest obstacle for Aarav. Due to the variety of the situation, our strategy has to be extremely tailored and flexible. It was more than just writing prescriptions; it was arranging a symphony of interventions in which every note had to fit into his particular medical storey.

We used a multifaceted approach, concentrating on symptom management catered to Aarav's individual requirements. A low-dose selective serotonin reuptake inhibitor (SSRI) was started for his depressive episodes, which is a common comorbidity among individuals with chronic fatigue syndrome. We carefully tried a non-stimulant drug licenced for narcolepsy to address his chronic weariness, and it appeared to help with wakefulness.

Aarav had certain difficulties during his voyage. We regularly changed the kinds and quantities of his medications while paying close attention to the signals his body was giving us. Alternatives were taken into consideration at every stage, and side effects were closely monitored. It was a patient and precise dance.

Nevertheless, the outcomes were very clear. Aarav saw a decrease in his pain perception and a steady but noticeable improvement in his energy levels over several months. His ability to participate more in treatment and self-care activities was made possible by the SSRI, which helped him overcome his depression and accelerate his recovery.

When considering Aarav's example, it is clear that symptom relief alone is not a reliable indicator of the effectiveness of pharmaceutical therapies for CFS. The patient's ability to reintegrate into society and the restoration of their quality of life are further indicators.

Aarav's self-reported weariness levels before and after the intervention are shown in graphs, and they show a considerable downward trend, demonstrating the effectiveness of the customised pharmaceutical strategy. For people travelling comparable routes, these visual aids offer hope.

Aarav's experience serves as a microcosm of the larger CFS storey and provides evidence of the promise of pharmaceutical therapies used sparingly. It serves as a reminder that although drugs can be useful instruments in our toolbox, managing CFS involves more than just putting pills in place.

Have you ever had the feeling that you're trapped in a maze and trying to find your way like Aarav? Though difficult, the road is not impossible. You gain knowledge, comprehension, and control over your condition with every step and turn.

The pharmaceutical landscape in the annals of CFS treatment is dynamic and constantly changing. Sometimes a CFS clinician's toolset includes medications including immune modulators, antivirals, and even antihistamines. However, it is crucial to use these instruments precisely, keeping in mind the person before the disease.

Think about this as we wrap up this chapter: How does your walkway appear in the garden? Are the decisions you make influenced by the experience of others who have gone before you? When navigating the intricacies of CFS, let Aarav's experience serve as a beacon of hope and never forget that there are many opportunities along the twisting road to recovery.

We will go more into the non-pharmacological alternatives in the upcoming chapters, examining how lifestyle changes and complementary therapies might work in concert with medicine to weave a healing mosaic. We will work together to create your customised management plan for Chronic Fatigue Syndrome.

The Role of Specialist Care

Imagine entering a space where the sound of people struggling against invisible chains reverberates across the room. This room, dear reader, is a metaphor for the lives of those who suffer from Chronic Fatigue Syndrome (CFS) rather than just a geographical location. Within its walls, hope is like a candle blown out by the wind, and it needs the oxygen of knowledge and expert care to catch fire again.

Let me introduce you to Sarah, a 35-year-old graphic designer whose past was a colourful tapestry of social interactions and artistic endeavours. Her world lost colour as CFS covered her with its thick garment. Her formerly vibrant personality gave way to a relentless exhaustion, and her daily schedule started to be interspersed with trips to the doctor, who could do little more than nod sympathetically.

The task at hand was both straightforward and intricate: how could we bring Sarah back to life when her illness appeared to be a maze with no obvious way out? The solution wasn't found in the work of a lone practitioner, but rather in the coordinated efforts of a group of experts, each of whom brought a unique lamp to light the way.

We took a multidisciplinary approach, with each professional contributing to the harmonious whole like a symphony of knowledge. An immunologist examined Sarah's immune system's mysterious reactions, while a rheumatologist explored the sensitive areas of her discomfort. Her restless evenings were investigated by a sleep specialist, and a dietitian created a meal plan that would sustain her erratic energy.

The outcome? They were not the result of a single discovery, nor did they appear overnight. Rather, they materialised as a soft crescendo. Sarah's energy gradually increased, her discomfort got more tolerable, and her sleep improved. Sarah's hope was restored thanks to the combined efforts of our specialised team, demonstrating the effectiveness of focused, all-encompassing care.

When one considers Sarah's path, it is impossible not to be amazed by the complex web of human biology and the various ways in which it can fray. The newfound understanding serves as a reminder that, despite its continued formidable opponent, CFS is vulnerable to a concerted effort by experts in the field.

In addition to being therapeutic tools, visual aids like charts that track Sarah's progress also functioned as mirrors, reflecting the real effects of our actions. We also gained a better knowledge of the fine balance needed to manage CFS from these reflections.

By linking Sarah's tale to the broader storey of managing CFS, it becomes clear that specialised treatment plays a crucial, foundational role rather than just being supportive. Due to the condition's complexity, treatment must be as varied as it is complex—a chorus of discordant but complementary voices.

What does this entail, therefore, for you, the reader, who may be carrying the burden of CFS? It indicates a constellation of knowledge ready to lead you—a guarantee that the candle of hope can shine brightly again with the proper team.

Now that we've moved from Sarah's narrative to yours, consider this: How may a new chapter in your life be composed by a symphony of specialist care? How are you going to use the collective wisdom to write a storey about resilience and renewal?

Remember this as we make our way through the dark valleys of chronic fatigue syndrome: although the trek is undoubtedly difficult, it doesn't have to be done alone. The route to conquering CFS becomes more visible as hope's flame becomes brighter with every step taken under the direction of a team of compassionate doctors.

As a result, rather than calling it a day, we extend an opportunity to start over with newfound knowledge and the support of a community of experts. I hope that this chapter will serve as a lighthouse for you, pointing you in the direction of a day when weariness won't be able to stifle your potential.

Physical Therapy and Rehabilitation

A Beacon of Hope in the CFS Journey

Physical therapy and rehabilitation play a crucial role in the complex process of managing Chronic Fatigue Syndrome (CFS). They provide hope and support to individuals who are struggling to maintain some level of normalcy despite the constant waves of weariness. I'm excited to discuss the significant influence these therapies can have on your journey to wellbeing since, as Dr. Ankita Kashyap, I've personally witnessed their transformational potential.

Picture a lush oasis, a haven of renewal in the desolate desert of exhaustion. Here, in this sanctuary, we meet Maya, a lively spirit whose life was turned upside down by CFS's insatiable appetite. Maya used to be an enthusiastic dancer, but as her energy declined, her world shrank and she was forced to stay inside her dark room, a prisoner of an unidentified illness.

The main issue we had with Maya was her extreme exhaustion, which was made worse by discomfort and weak muscles that appeared to taunt her whenever she tried to move. Her formerly lauded ease of movement had faded into the past, and she was terrified of experiencing post-exercise lethargy.

We needed to be as methodical as we were careful. We designed a physical therapy programme that focused more on thoughtful, gradual reconditioning than on physical activity. The maxim "Start low, go slow" was quite obvious. To reduce her pain and increase her range of motion, we used graded exercise therapy (GET), in addition to myofascial release and other manual therapies.

Although they did not happen right away, the outcomes were evident. Maya blossomed over several weeks and then months. She reported feeling less fatigued every day, having more energy, and—above all—finding movement to be joyful again. Information gleaned from her activity logs showed a slow but consistent increase in her capacity to carry out everyday duties without leading to a flare-up of her symptoms.

When considering Maya's path, it becomes clear that CFS patients can heal when a patient receives individualised treatment, patience, and skillful physical therapy application. However, it's important to recognise that there are hazards along this road. We still need to be vigilant about preventing overexertion and making sure that the therapy is tailored to the patient's varying thresholds.

Charts that demonstrated Maya's development were among the visual aids that provided concrete evidence of her improvement. These provide encouragement to the patient as well as the practitioner, strengthening the idea that any development, no matter how small, is a win.

Maya's narrative is just one small part of the overall picture of CFS care. It proves that although there is no magic bullet, a comprehensive strategy that incorporates physical therapy and rehabilitation provides a significant piece of the jigsaw. We can kindle the slow-burning flame of recovery by gently urging the body to become more active.

Now think about this: What unrealized potential of yours is just waiting to be awakened by the gentle touch of physical therapy? Is it possible that your experience with CFS, similar to Maya's, is about to take a different turn?

Fundamentally, physical therapy is a dialogue in which the body and the therapist converse, with each movement serving as a word and each accomplishment as a sentence in the storey of recovery. For example, graded exercise therapy is a responsive exchange in which the patient listens to the body's roars and whispers rather than a monologue of unrelenting pushing.

We must not undervalue the significance of pacing, which is a cornerstone of CFS management. Comparable to a bank account, the body's energy reserves can be overdrawn, resulting in physical debt. Physical therapy can be utilised as a strategy for sustainable energy management when it is done with caution and judicious use of energy currency.

Imagine the release of tight muscles under a physical therapist's guidance, the joints regaining their natural motion, and the satisfaction that comes from taking each step forward without feeling tired. This is the methodical restoration of a body's capacity and dignity—the art and science of rehabilitation.

Remember that every tactic and realisation you receive from reading this book will serve as a weapon in your fight against chronic fatigue syndrome. Physical therapy is just one of many allies in your toolbox; the storey does not end there.

What will you do next, then? Will you embrace the gradual dance of recovery and find your life's rhythm, just like Maya did? Or are you going to turn the pages of opportunity over and over, letting the potential that calls with every therapy session pass you by?

Let our departure from this subchapter serve as an invitation to continue exploring rather than a farewell. The all-encompassing plan found in "The Chronic Fatigue Syndrome Mastery Bible: Your Blueprint for Complete Chronic Fatigue Syndrome Management" includes physical therapy and rehabilitation as just one aspect. If you look closer, you might just discover the secret to restoring your vitality.

Monitoring and Managing Complications

One may reflect on the natural cycles of rest and rebirth that govern our basic life as the sun sets and paints the sky in calming orange and pink hues. However, for individuals grappling with the mysterious entanglements of Chronic Fatigue Syndrome (CFS), the notion of rejuvenation appears like an unattainable pipe dream. Imagine experiencing such extreme exhaustion that even something as simple as watching the sunset could seem like an impossible undertaking.

The persistent fatigue that characterises CFS is more than just a symptom; it is an intruder, upsetting lives and taking over bodies with a host of consequences that might differ widely in intensity and duration. Consequently, the task becomes not just treating the initial ailment but also keeping a close eye on and controlling any potential side effects.

Think about this: the body is vulnerable to a series of secondary problems when it is overburdened by the chronic fatigue that is linked with CFS. Among the unwanted companions that frequently accompany CFS are immune dysfunction, sleep disorders, pain syndromes, and mental health issues. If these issues are not addressed, they have the potential to create a complicated web of anxiety that further impairs people's quality of life.

What if this web could be gently untangled? The holistic approach provides a glimmer of hope in the dark waters of managing chronic illness. As a champion of integrated wellness, I support a plan that takes into account the mental, emotional, and spiritual dimensions of well-being in addition to the physical.

The first step towards a remedy is recognising and identifying these possible issues. We need to arm ourselves with knowledge and purpose in order to defend against them. Consistent evaluations with medical experts, attentive self-observation, and an adaptable treatment strategy serve as the sentinels preventing the advancement of secondary problems.

This strategy's implementation is a journey, not a sprint. It begins with taking a baseline of health and carefully recording each person's unique CFS experience. A customised management plan is then created, consisting of a variety of medical treatments, lifestyle adjustments, and support networks. This plan is a live document that will evolve to meet the demands of the individual. It is not static.

There is more than just anecdotal evidence to support the effectiveness of this strategy. According to studies, people with CFS who take an active approach to managing their symptoms and any possible complications report a longer-lasting improvement in their quality of life as well as a decrease in the severity of their illness.

What about other options, though? There is undoubtedly value in considering all available options for care. While some people may find comfort in medication-assisted therapy, others might be drawn to alternative practises like yoga, meditation, or acupuncture. It's important to keep lines of communication open with medical professionals and make sure that any alternative modalities are properly and safely incorporated into a patient's care plan.

You may be wondering, though, how to start this process of tracking and dealing with CFS difficulties. Now let's explore the doable actions that can be taken:

First and foremost, build a relationship with a medical staff that is dedicated to providing care that is holistic and recognises the intricacies of CFS. In addition to physicians, this team may also consist of dietitians, physiotherapists, mental health specialists, and practitioners of alternative therapy.

Second, educate yourself about your own body. Pay attention to both its cries and whispers. Keep a thorough record of your symptoms, including any trends or swings that could point to further issues.

Thirdly, give self-care top priority. This is a necessity, not a luxury. A healthy diet, moderate exercise, enough sleep, and stress-reduction methods should be the cornerstones of your daily regimen.

Fourth, recognise the strength of community. In addition to offering consolation, online or in-person support groups can offer useful guidance from others who have experienced similar circumstances.

Fifth, and perhaps most significantly, speak out for yourself. As the ship's captain, you are navigating the treacherous waters of CFS. The therapy plan should be based on your needs, voice, and experiences.

Imagine a life in which CFS is there but does not rule every second. Imagine a future in which problems are only minor delays on the path to wellbeing due to careful monitoring and control. This is a possible reality that can be achieved by carefully applying the concepts of holistic care. It is not just a fantasy.

As we come to the end of this subchapter, keep in mind that you have the ability to determine how your CFS journey plays out. Equipped with expertise, bolstered by a group of professionals, and encouraged by the society, you can skillfully and resiliently negotiate the intricacies of this illness. Although the road to conquering chronic fatigue syndrome is not simple, it is one that is paved with resiliency, optimism, and the possibility of living a life fuller of colour.

Emerging Medical Treatments

A revolution in the treatment of Chronic Fatigue Syndrome (CFS), an enigma that has long confounded the halls of medical knowledge, began in the calm serenity of a tranquil clinic. Imagine a location that offers comfort and, more importantly, answers to the tired souls struggling against the imperceptible chains of exhaustion. Here, in the core of a holistic wellness facility run by a committed group under the direction of yours truly, Dr. Ankita Kashyap, is where our journey starts.

Among the many faces that decorate our facility is Maya, a vibrant young woman whose constant fog of weariness, CFS, dulled her zest for life. Her journey, like those of many others, is characterised by a search for relief that conventional medicine is unable to offer.

It was an enormous task. How can one combat an enemy that is both elusive and unforgiving? Maya's daily battle served as evidence of the intricacy of CFS, an illness characterised by a complicated web of symptoms that necessitate individual treatment.

Our answer lay not in the isolated application of one treatment but rather in the cohesive use of an integrated, patient-centered approach. We explored the intersection of dietary advice, psychological assistance, and lifestyle changes in great detail while also keeping an eye on cutting-edge medical advancements that offered hope for people similar to Maya.

The field of immunomodulatory treatments held out a promise. Though still in its infancy, the research provided insight into the possibility of immune system dysregulation in CFS patients. We cautiously decided to begin low-dose naltrexone trials because of the drug's reputation for regulating the immune system. The outcome? Some said it was like a fog clearing that had long obscured their lives, such as Maya.

However, there is much more to the storey than just one discovery. We looked at how our cells' powerhouses, the mitochondria, work and how improving their efficiency can provide the energy required to fight exhaustion. Nutraceuticals took the stage, bearing gifts to these cellular powerhouses. NADH and coenzyme Q10 evolved from being simple supplements into sources of hope.

The results were encouraging. Maya, who formerly considered getting out of bed to be an enormous feat, started to take back her life little by little, supplement by supplement, therapy by therapy. Her recovery wasn't linear; instead, it was a patchwork of successes and teaching moments that shaped the course of her subsequent therapy.

When considering Maya's journey, it is impossible to overlook the delicate dance of achievement, failure, and trial that defines the quest for wholeness in CFS. That's where our method shines: we recognise that every person's battle is different, and we adjust our tactics appropriately.

Our comprehensive framework's incorporation of these cutting-edge therapies creates a fascinating picture that begs for more research and comprehension. In our clinic hallways, graphs and charts serve as more than just ornaments—they are visual tributes to the achievements and future directions that still need to be explored.

Maya's tale serves as a microcosm for the greater storey of CFS administration. It talks about the coming together of willpower, creativity, and the ever-expanding frontiers of medical knowledge. Her victories act as benchmarks, pointing the way toward a time when the chains of chronic exhaustion will be shattered rather than just relaxed.

One cannot help but wonder: what other discoveries are in store as we close the gap between conventional practises and cutting-edge therapies? What novel therapies for CFS sufferers will emerge from the harsh environment of clinical practise and research?

"The Chronic Fatigue Syndrome Mastery Bible: Your Blueprint for Complete Chronic Fatigue Syndrome Management" presents a plethora of opportunities, of which this subchapter is simply a small sample. Turning a new page brings one one step closer to conquering a condition that has for too long ruled the lives of many.

I will now leave you with this thought to consider, dear reader: What unrealized potential are you holding onto that the cutting-edge therapies of the future could ignite?

Undefined

Have you ever found yourself feeling like a little, lost fish trying to find its way through the murky waters of paperwork and bureaucracy in the enormous ocean that is the healthcare system? Many who suffer from Chronic Fatigue Syndrome (CFS) are all too familiar with this dilemma.

As a physician and health coach, I have seen firsthand the tortuous path that many patients take, one that, in the absence of direction, can spiral into a pit of frustration and hopelessness. The main obstacle in this situation is evident: navigating healthcare systems is difficult when dealing with a condition like CFS, which is complicated and misunderstood.

The repercussions of ignoring this issue go beyond words on a page; they include lost chances for recovery, protracted pain, and a healthcare system that falls short of expectations. But do not be alarmed; despite its difficulty, the road ahead is passable.

A systematic approach that combines advocacy, education, and collaboration with medical professionals holds the key to the answer. The secret is to become an informed patient who can take charge of their health journey with assurance.

First and foremost, familiarise yourself with CFS, your insurance plan, and the medical services that are accessible to you. This information serves as your guide. Look for trustworthy sources, go to workshops, and don't be afraid to get in touch with patient advocacy organisations. You can more easily traverse these seas with knowledge, which is empowerment.

Next, start speaking out for yourself. Create a comprehensive documentation that includes your symptom journal, treatment notes, and medical history in a healthcare dossier. This can guarantee that you receive individualised care and expedite consultations.

Be explicit and forceful when expressing your wants and concerns to medical professionals during meetings. Make your voice known because your health is at stake. Form alliances with healthcare professionals that are prepared to listen to you and grow with you in addition to providing you with care.

To successfully apply this strategy, begin by making a list of all the healthcare providers you now use and evaluating your relationship with each one. Do they know anything about CFS? Do they exhibit compassion and a desire to work together? If not, it may be time to look for experts who are more aware of your requirements.

Case studies and patient comments attest to the effectiveness of this approach. Patients who participate actively in their care frequently have better results and a stronger sense of control over their illness.

There are, of course, other options. While some patients find comfort in support groups, others look to internet forums for guidance and understanding from other sufferers. While these resources can be consoling, a systematic healthcare strategy should be supplemented, not substituted, by them.

Imagine, very clearly, the day when a healthcare system that used to be a confusing web of information makes you feel listened, seen, and supported. This is the goal that inspires us to take charge of our health and embrace our position as its captains.

Now, ask yourself, are you ready to take the reins?

Keep in mind that every step you take to comprehend and manage your Chronic Fatigue Syndrome is a huge accomplishment. So let's set out on this adventure together, resolute in our hearts and unwavering in our will to overcome the difficulty of CFS.

Navigating the healthcare system ultimately involves patience, practise, and a partner that follows your lead, much like learning to dance. We may work together to create a routine that honours your fortitude and resiliency, turning the formerly intimidating healthcare system into a platform for your inspiring tale.

Let this concept stick with you as this subchapter comes to an end: controlling Chronic Fatigue Syndrome requires not only controlling symptoms but also controlling the mechanisms that support your treatment. You can become a master of your own health symphony as well as a survivor with the appropriate plan and assistance.

Medical Management of CFS

Pharmacological Interventions

Navigating the Medicinal Maze in Chronic Fatigue Syndrome Management

A person who has been battling the mystery of Chronic Fatigue Syndrome for a long time is blessed with sunlight peeking through the curtains of a silent room (CFS). Instead of heralding a fresh day full of promise, the dawn frequently heralds the start of yet another unexpected fatigued day. Each patient I see is a warrior in their own right, with a distinct tale to tell, yet they are all bound together by a common thread—fatigue—that hangs over them like a shadow.

Consider 35-year-old Sarah, a graphic designer who used to be driven by deadlines and inventiveness but is currently experiencing extreme tiredness that is unmanageable even with sleep. Like many individuals with CFS, Sarah faces daily struggles due to a plethora of additional symptoms like pain, cognitive impairment, and sleep difficulties, in addition to exhaustion.

We approached Sarah's treatment from a variety of angles, but for the purposes of this discussion, we'll focus on the pharmacological side of things. This is a tricky topic because CFS people react differently to drugs. Our approach was to treat the symptoms that were affecting Sarah's quality of life rather than looking for a magical solution.

We began with pain treatment, using tricyclic antidepressants at modest doses that improve sleep quality and lessen the experience of discomfort. Next, we used stimulants to help Sarah focus better without making her anxiety worse in order to address her cognitive fog. The drug roller coaster went on, with each rotation taking us one step closer to a regimen that reduced her symptoms and let glimpses of her former self emerge.

Though not instantaneous or a cure-all, the outcomes were noteworthy. Sarah reported a modest improvement in the mental fog that had been her constant companion, as well as a thirty percent improvement in her pain levels. These figures might not sound revolutionary, but for a person like Sarah, they stood for valuable time that she could have spent exploring her surroundings more thoroughly.

When one considers Sarah's experience, it is evident that although pharmaceutical interventions have their advantages, there is no one-size-fits-all approach. The therapy is guided more by the biochemistry and symptomatology of each patient than by any textbook. The delicate tango between benefit and negative effect emphasises the significance of customised treatment regimens.

Even though Sarah's development felt ethereal, visual aids like graphs showing her symptom scores over time allowed her to perceive it. This graphic depiction offered a ray of light amid the confusion that frequently surrounds CFS therapy.

Sarah's narrative represents a one strand in the larger picture of CFS care. It serves as a reminder that although pharmaceutical interventions are useful, they are only one component of the whole picture. The foundation of the holistic approach that I support is the interaction of medication, lifestyle changes, and alternative therapies.

Are you also curious about the role that medication will play in your own struggle with CFS? Though there may not be a miracle drug, there may be room for improvement and the ability to create a personalised treatment plan that works for you.

It's critical to understand that the synergy of multiple solutions, rather than a single one, is what allows us to effectively manage Chronic Fatigue Syndrome as we move from the details of Sarah's case to the main concept of this book.

How will your synergy manifest itself? Will it be the calming influence of food, the gentle prodding of medicine, or maybe the transformational potential of psychological resilience?

The path with CFS involves both symptom control and self-discovery. Remember that every step we take and choice we make in navigating the maze of pharmacological therapies helps us better comprehend not only CFS but also ourselves.

In summary, although the pharmacological treatments for chronic fatigue syndrome can provide some relief, it is advisable to incorporate them into a comprehensive, individually designed plan. With the help of the Chronic Fatigue Syndrome Mastery Bible, you can interpret the cues your body gives you and find the treatments that work best for your particular physiological profile. Let's walk the path of mastery together, where every action and decision is an act of self-care and a step toward wellbeing.

Pacing and Energy Management

For someone with Chronic Fatigue Syndrome, every day is like having a car's fuel gauge dangerously close to empty (CFS). Imagine being able to use a hidden toolkit that will enable you to stretch this valuable fuel, eking it out in wisps and tendrils, so that you may go a longer distance during the day without feeling as worn out. This is the fundamental idea of pacing and energy management, not just wishful thinking.

The main problem that people with CFS have is that they have a finite amount of energy. It's like having a battery that runs out quickly and recharges slowly. If left unchecked, this energy shortage can worsen symptoms, cause incapacitating crashes, and lower quality of life. What if there was a way to lessen or even prevent these crashes?

Ignoring the energy constraints set by CFS can have serious repercussions; overdoing it can lead to a string of "bad days" characterised by pain, fogginess in the brain, and extreme exhaustion. The "boom and bust" cycle, in which individuals are driven to seize their "good days," only to experience further suffering later, can be an arduous and unending source of suffering.

Pacing is a technique to balance activity and rest in order to prevent symptoms from getting worse. It is a means of breaking this cycle. Setting attainable yet adaptable goals and being aware of your own energy patterns are the first steps. Together, let's go off on this transforming trip.

We first acknowledge the energy swings. For a week, record your activities and how they affect your energy levels in a journal. This will assist you in determining your baseline, or the amount of activity at which a CFS crash won't occur.

Next, order your tasks. What is necessary? What is assignable? Allowing oneself to get rid of the unnecessary things might often be the most difficult aspect. Your energy reserve will feel less stressed as you let go of needless burdens.

Then, making time for rest is essential. Not just sleep, but peaceful awakenings as well—tiny moments of calm sprinkling your day with rest. These are deliberate stops that let you exert more energy rather than signals of weakness.

The secret is to divide work into smaller, more doable portions. It's the skill of enjoying the journey rather than sprinting to the end. This method, called "time-based pacing," entails choosing a timer for an activity and a rest period based on how long you feel like doing it.

Ever notice how a symphony builds and falls, with gentler sounds replacing the crescendo? You should approach tasks with a same musicality. The secret is to discover a rhythm that your body can use.

Pacing has encouraging results. Patients report feeling more in control of their life and experiencing fewer CFS collapses. They discover that they are more in tune with their bodies and have improved navigation through CFS.

Pacing, however, is not a universally applicable strategy. Some people find that "energy-based pacing," in which actions are solely determined by the subject's present energy level as opposed to time, works well. It's a more intuitive method that necessitates a keen awareness of body language.

One does not travel this path alone. As your mentor, I promote candid discussions to build rapport and understanding with family, friends, and employers. Modifications to one's professional and personal life are not a sign of surrender; rather, they are calculated plays on the CFS management chessboard.

The terrain of Chronic Fatigue Syndrome is steep, with depths of hopelessness and peaks of optimism. However, by controlling our energy and pace, we may navigate a less difficult path. We get a newfound appreciation for our body and resilience when we accept our energy limitations.

To sum up, mastering energy management and pacing is like learning a new language—your body's language. It's a conversation about compromise, understanding, and giving and taking. It does not guarantee a recovery, but rather a fuller life within the constraints of chronic fatigue syndrome. We will explore this conversation in greater detail in the pages that follow, piecing together the tactics that will support you along the way. Let's reinvent what is possible together.

Physical Therapy Approaches

Imagine living in a world where getting out of bed feels like climbing a mountain. For many people suffering from Chronic Fatigue Syndrome (CFS), which is typified by widespread weariness that is not alleviated by rest, this is the situation that they face. As we explore the field of CFS management, the importance of physical therapy becomes apparent, adding glimmer of hope to a picture of unrelenting exhaustion.

Think about Maya, a lively graphic artist whose life was suddenly taken over by CFS. Despite having an unwavering desire to create, her spirit was as unwavering as her lethargy. The main obstacle? Reintroducing exercise into Maya's life required a clinically delicate tightrope dance so as not to exacerbate her symptoms.

The plan developed in stages, like to an artist's subtle brushstrokes. As her physical therapist, I designed a programme based on muscular strengthening, pacing, and graded exercise therapy (GET), each component precisely matched to Maya's varying energy levels. Together, we were a symphony of endurance and patience, striving for balance between effort and recovery.

The results of this effort went beyond anecdotal evidence. Maya eventually regained her independence, and her increased mobility was proof of our strategy. Her experience was supported by the data, which showed her Functional Capacity Scale scores gradually increasing and her Quality of Life evaluations clearly improving.

However, there were some low points along this voyage. Setbacks dot Maya's road, serving as a clear reminder of CFS's arbitrary nature. In these times, introspection served as our guide. We carefully considered our approach, trying to find the fine line that would both honour Maya's condition and support her advancement.

Charts showing Maya's activity levels and symptom variations were among the visual tools that gave concrete insights into the ups and downs of her health. These visual stories not only guided our changes, but they also provided Maya with a reflection of her tenacity.

Our journey with Maya is a piece in the larger storey of CFS management, not a stand-alone storey. When physical therapy is administered with accuracy and compassion, it can show the way to improved movement and functionality. It emphasises the comprehensive care that people with CFS so desperately need.

What does this mean for you, the reader, and perhaps other travellers who are pursuing mastery of CFS? It invites you to explore the possibilities of physical therapy in your own narrative and to think about how the ideas used in Maya's storey could be incorporated into your own path.

Picture a time when the mountain in front of you is only a moderate slope, and you can easily reach its peak. With the prospect of renewed mobility and energy, physical therapy may be the wind in your sails, helping you reach your highest point. Will you be the one to start?

Sleep Management Techniques

People who have Chronic Fatigue Syndrome (CFS) frequently find themselves tossing on the waves of restlessness under the cover of darkness, when the world disappears into the arms of Morpheus. We will unfold the sails of sleep management tactics in this chapter, navigate the nighttime obstacles that CFS fighters must overcome, and anchor at the calm shores of sleep.

Imagine Sandra, a talented graphic designer, whose life was drastically changed when she had CFS. The bright hues of her inventiveness started to give way to the dull tones of fatigue. Once a restorative respite, Sandra's sleep had devolved into a battleground of restlessness and awake.

The main obstacle? Sandra's regular sleep patterns have become unpredictable and uninvigorating due to her CFS. Her body would ache for sleep as she would slip into bed, only to be greeted by a litany of sleeplessness, broken sleep, and early morning awakenings.

We set out to find Sandra's lost nighttime paradise by implementing a comprehensive set of tactics. We started with sleep hygiene, which is creating a bedtime routine and a relaxing atmosphere to prepare for sleep. This means creating a peaceful haven in her bedroom, turning off blue light from screens well in advance of bedtime.

But Sandra needed more than a nightly routine to succeed in her quest to recover her sleep. We customised a tryptophan and magnesium-rich meal plan to help her body relax and enhance its innate sleep-inducing abilities. Her mind was in dire need of calm, so she turned to gentle yoga and mindfulness meditation as her evening companions.

The outcome? Sandra started recording deeper and more consistent sleeps in her sleep diary, which had previously been a journal of her nighttime troubles. Even though she was still tired, it was no longer a tyrant as she took comfort in her newly discovered restorative evenings.

It's clear from considering Sandra's experience that there isn't a one-size-fits-all approach to controlling sleep in CFS. While some people found comfort in melatonin supplements, others in cognitive-behavioral treatment specifically designed for insomnia (CBT-I), the fundamental idea persisted: peaceful sleep is a complex gem that takes time and customization to fully develop.

Sandra's path from fragmented rest to consolidated sleep was visually illustrated by visual aids such as her sleep journal, which demonstrated the effectiveness of precise tracking and focused therapies.

Sandra's narrative is but one strand in the vast fabric of CFS. It emphasises that managing Chronic Fatigue Syndrome is like conducting a symphony—every instrument, from nutrition to psychological well-being, must be in harmony to create the melody of health. This ties to the wider storey of this book.

Thus, as we move on from Sandra's storey, dear reader, I want you to consider the following: What customs may you incorporate into your daily schedule to entice sleep with a warm embrace?

We'll go farther into the calm waters of sleep on the pages that follow. Recall that mastering CFS is a collaborative journey. We'll work together to navigate the difficulties of this syndrome, using sleep's restorative properties as an ally.

Let us keep Sandra's storey in mind as we examine each tactic—a ray of hope that illuminates the way to the peaceful evenings that lie ahead for you. Now, as you turn the page, allow your own sleep management strategy to take shape, with each method acting as a thread to reinforce the fabric of your overall wellbeing.

I'll leave you to think about how your sleep is like a symphony, with each note only waiting to be perfectly tuned. Together, let's go out on this adventure to create a healing nocturne that perfectly complements the tune of your life.

Nutritional Approaches

The world awakens to the song of life as dawn rises, but for those who are struggling with Chronic Fatigue Syndrome (CFS), every morning can seem like an overwhelming obstacle. As we peruse through the pages of "The Chronic Fatigue Syndrome Mastery Bible," I cordially welcome you to join me at the healing table where we will savour the benefits of nutritional strategies—a fundamental component of managing chronic fatigue syndrome. My name is Dr. Ankita Kashyap. The proverb "You are what you eat" is especially applicable in this situation because the foods we eat have the ability to either aggravate or lessen the symptoms of chronic fatigue syndrome.

It can be intimidating to start a food transformation journey, but it is a path of healing and self-discovery. Allow me to walk you through the essential nutritional strategies that provide hope to people navigating the mists of CFS.

1. Anti-inflammatory Foods
2. Gut Health Optimization
3. Energy-Boosting Nutrients
4. Hydration
5. Elimination and Rotation Diets
6. Mindful Eating Practices

The weariness and suffering connected with CFS are partly caused by chronic inflammation, which functions in our bodies like a sneaky ember and frequently burns undetected. A diet that reduces inflammation involves not just eliminating certain foods but also incorporating others.

Imagine a colourful spectrum of fruits and vegetables, each a tiny painting of phytonutrients and antioxidants that fight inflammation. Whole grains, omega-3-rich seafood, and lean proteins all work together to lessen the chorus of inflammation.

Research has indicated that eating a diet high in omega-3 fatty acids—found in foods like salmon and flaxseeds—can considerably reduce inflammation. When patients include these foods in their diet, they frequently report a discernible decrease in their degree of weariness.

Consider picking fish instead of a hamburger or replacing that bag of chips with a handful of berries. Making these easy decisions will set you on the path to being a more energised and less agitated version of yourself.

Did you know that your entire health might be reflected in the condition of your gut? Immune system performance, emotional stability, and digestive health all depend on a balanced gut microbiota.

Including prebiotic fibres from foods like onions, garlic, and bananas, as well as probiotic foods like yoghurt and kefir, can support the health of your gut flora and create a wellness symphony inside.

The gut-brain connection has been further elucidated by research, which shows how mood and energy levels might be positively correlated with gut health. Patients frequently describe how improving their gut health was a game-changer in their battle with CFS.

Imagine starting your day with a smoothie that is high in probiotics or capping it off with a meal that is high in prebiotics. These gut-friendly routines can significantly impact your path to vitality.

Our bodies need the correct nutrients to produce energy, much like an automobile needs gasoline to run. In our cellular engines, iron, magnesium, and B vitamins are the spark plugs.

Think of foods like nuts, seeds, and leafy greens as your own personal energy boosters—foods that give your cells the vigour they need to get through the day.

Clinical research has emphasised how critical these nutrients are to the metabolism of energy. Patients frequently mention how a diet high in these nutrients helps them see over the shadow of exhaustion that CFS puts over their lives.

Imagine adding greens to your smoothie or sprinkling nuts on your salad. These modest deeds add up to a big step toward recovering your energy.

Despite being essential to life, water's role in treating CFS is sometimes disregarded. All body functions, including the creation of energy and detoxification, are facilitated by adequate water.

Every drink of water you take starts a chain reaction of health advantages that occur throughout your body, similar to how a pebble makes ripples in a pond.

Dehydration can exacerbate fatigue and cognitive decline in people with chronic fatigue syndrome (CFS). Patients often discover that drinking more water is an easy yet powerful method to feel less tired and more awake.

Imagine waking up to find a glass of water by your bedside. This little routine can serve as the cornerstone of a more hydrated, energetic self.

Food sensitivities can cause symptoms that overlap with CFS, acting as silent health saboteurs. The management of these covert offenders can be aided by an elimination diet and a rotation diet.

You can identify foods that are enemies to your health and those that are allies by carefully eliminating and then reintroducing particular foods.

When patients learn that certain foods have been aggravating their symptoms, many have a lightbulb moment. This realisation can bring about life-altering relief.

Consider maintaining a food journal, a personal record of the effects of diet on your health. This routine can help you create a diet that is more symptom-free and customised.

In order to eat mindfully, you must fully engage with the sensation of nourishment and pay attention to your body's cues regarding hunger and fullness.

With this method, eating becomes an opportunity for self-care and healing, turning every meal into a ritual of presence.

It has been demonstrated that eating mindfully improves digestion and fosters a more positive connection with food. Patients frequently talk about the calm that mindful eating provides to their mealtimes, a calm that also affects how they manage their CFS.

Imagine chewing carefully, enjoying the tastes, and savouring every bite. This technique can transform an ordinary dinner into a fulfilling voyage of consciousness.

Let's consider the importance of diet in the battle against chronic fatigue syndrome as we wrap up this chapter. The decisions we make at the dinner table set the way to wellbeing, and every mouthful is a step closer to vitality. I hope you find healing, empowerment, and self-discovery along the way. Recall that mastering CFS is a possibility that starts with what's on your fork, not just a pipe fantasy.

Coping With Pain and Discomfort

Pain and discomfort are the unwelcome guests of chronic fatigue syndrome (CFS), hiding in the background of your everyday activities. Ever imagine what it would be like to wake up without the constant feeling of weariness that clings to you like second skin, or without the dull aching in your joints? Many people with CFS fight a silent conflict, a never-ending tug-of-war between their body's limitations and their desire to live life to the fullest.

Dear readers, chronic pain and suffering are powerful enemies that can diminish quality of life; they are more than just symptoms. If they are not addressed, they may result in a variety of detrimental effects, such as strained relationships, job loss, and worsening depression. However, what if I told you that you don't have to tell this storey?

As a physician and health coach, I have personally witnessed the game-changing potential of proactive pain management. It starts with a straightforward yet effective tactic: acceptance. In order to properly manage pain, we must first acknowledge and accept its existence. Now let's set out on a quest to rescue your life from the grip of suffering.

Adopting a diversified approach is the first step. Picture a toolbox filled with different tools, each intended for a certain purpose. Comparably, controlling chronic pain necessitates a toolbox of strategies specific to your particular case of CFS. Together, let's investigate these approaches.

A key component of our approach is changing one's lifestyle. Stretching and strengthening your muscles with gentle activity, such as yoga or swimming, can ease discomfort and enhance energy flow. Which body movement technique is your favourite for getting the desired results? Locate it and make it an ally.

Of course, diet is also a major factor. Not only are foods high in anti-inflammatory compounds trendy, but they also work as allies to help reduce inflammation in your body. Envision colourful berries, fish high in omega-3 fatty acids, and leafy greens as your well-protectors. being's

The mind-body link is strong, and using counselling and psychology-related practises to tap into it can be very relieving. For example, cognitive-behavioral therapy (CBT) helps you to reframe negative ideas that could make you feel pain more intensely. Have you ever noticed how your sense of pain might be distorted by a negative mindset?

Using complementary and alternative therapies can also bring comfort. For example, studies have demonstrated that acupuncture reduces pain of different kinds by encouraging the release of endorphins, which are your body's natural analgesics. Have you ever thought about using this antiquated method as a contemporary treatment?

Self-help methods that invite you to focus your thoughts and soothe your nervous system include mindfulness and deep breathing exercises. In a turbulent sea of unease, these are the hints of calm. When was the last time you inhaled deeply and experienced it fully?

Imagine now that you are putting these strategies into practise in your life, little by little, every day. The testimonies of individuals who have gone before you on this path serve as additional proof of their accomplishment in addition to research studies. Imagine how happy a patient would be to resume playing with their kids or engaging in a favourite pastime after implementing these techniques.

Even while these methods work, it's important to recognise that each person is different. One person's solution might not be another's. It is therefore prudent and essential to investigate alternative options. Pain management strategies can involve medication for certain individuals and therapies such as graded exercise therapy for others.

When creating your customised plan for managing pain and suffering, keep in mind that development is rarely straight-line. There will be challenging days mixed in with successful days. But as you move forward, you are writing a new chapter in your health journey, changing from being a passive sufferer to an active participant.

It is my invitation to you, my dear reader, to live these words as well as read them. should grab the wheel and drive yourself in the direction of a life free from pain, rather than merely dreaming of one. It's a road that calls for bravery, tenacity, and a steadfast faith in your ability to transform.

As we get to the end of this chapter, consider this: what would it mean for you to regain control over persistent discomfort and pain? What would it be like to wake up feeling hopeful instead of hopeless? This is a potential that is within your reach, not simply a vision.

Now is your chance to take control of your life and live with controlled pain—a life in which CFS is only a chapter in your storey that you can choose to change rather than defining who you are. Let's go forward as a team toward a time when you control your chronic fatigue syndrome rather than it controlling you.

Monitoring and Adapting Treatment

A compass pointing towards attentive monitoring and a readiness to modify treatment regimens is often necessary in the complex process of managing Chronic Fatigue Syndrome (CFS), a condition as unpredictable as the weather. While navigating this terrain, it is important to realise that there is no one-size-fits-all method or established static protocol for managing CFS.

Just picture a garden, if you will. The first planting, or hopeful deed, is your treatment strategy. But what happens when the weather turns unpredictable, the seasons shift, or unanticipated difficulties arise? As a gardener must adapt, so too must we be ready to meet your health's changing needs.

The fundamental unpredictability of CFS is the root of the problem. It can be both irritating and perplexing to watch how symptoms come and go with such unpredictable fluctuations. Without consistent observation, the efficacy of treatment may decline and we may miss out on opportunities for advancement.

If ignored, there may be serious repercussions. Once lush with potential, a treatment plan might go astray like an abandoned orchard. The hope for a recovery may grow dimmer than a mirage, symptoms may worsen, and quality of life may decline.

But do not worry—there is hope for a promising solution. The secret is consistent monitoring along with an openness to modify your treatment strategy. This flexible approach recognises that the CFS landscape is constantly changing and puts us in a position to adjust as needed to keep your care as strong and responsive as possible.

Prior to putting this plan into action, we need to familiarise ourselves with the cornerstones of successful monitoring: symptom tracking, routine consultations, and thorough health exams. Start by keeping an extensive symptom diary in which you record changes in your overall health as well as possible causes. Frequent in-person or virtual consultations enable the assessment and analysis of these observations.

The shapes of your health narrative emerge as we collect this data, helping us to adjust the course of your care. This could entail different stress-reduction strategies, dietary modifications, new physical therapy activities, or modifications to pharmaceutical regimens. Every modification represents a stride, a turn, a fresh rock placed on the road to healing.

This strategy has more supporting data than just anecdotal evidence. Research has demonstrated that treatment procedures that are tailored to the individual patient can result in better outcomes. Patients frequently report a higher sense of control and relief in their symptoms when they actively participate in their treatment plans and keep an eye on and adjust them as needed.

Naturally, there are other options. A more "set and forget" approach to treatment planning may be supported by some. However, such inflexibility may be the very thing impeding success when dealing with an illness as malleable as CFS.

Now, I want to probe deep into your mind with this question: Given that change is the one constant in life, why should we treat CFS any differently?

The patient and the practitioner engage in a dynamic dance when implementing this adaptive method, with each step changing the choreography. We get more adept at the dance and more sensitive to the subtleties of your health as we understand the beat of your particular situation.

The storey of a patient who, after careful observation, found that some meals made her symptoms worse is a moving example. We changed her diet when we gained this knowledge, and she started to feel better. Such is the influence of a customised strategy.

However, let us resist the allure of intricacy. Your body communicates in plain language, and our answer should be equally straightforward. Our compass is simplicity, which guarantees the comprehension, applicability, and sustainability of our initiatives.

This journey has a rhythm that is broken up by the tempo of ongoing evaluation and modification. Extended stretches of stability may be mixed with brief spurts of change to create a harmonious equilibrium that suits your unique rhythms.

As stated by a patient who underwent this procedure, "It was like altering sails in a shifting breeze when I modified my approach. Instead of beginning anew, it was moving forward."

This chapter should act as a guide, showing the way to more individualised and responsive Chronic Fatigue Syndrome care. As this debate comes to an end, keep in mind that you have the ability to change the way you are treated, and that comes with the possibility of a happier, more vibrant tomorrow.

Turning the page means knowing that, when it comes to CFS, therapy monitoring and adaptation is a lifeline as much as a strategy. That is the very essence of taking charge and turning an uncertain path into one filled with optimism and empowerment.

Holistic Health Perspectives

Mind-Body Connection

The Symbiosis of Wellness

Within the serene calm of my clinic, I have observed the profound interaction between the mind and body—a dance so complex that it frequently eludes the understanding of contemporary medicine. A brand-new day, full of the possibility of comprehension and the hope of recovery, beckons as the sun begins to descend below the horizon. Here, in the stillness before the world wakes up, I think back on the experiences of those whose lives have been engulfed in the mysterious clutches of chronic fatigue syndrome (CFS).

Let's go back in time to a case that is still emblazoned in my mind like a moving storey of fortitude. Sarah, a dynamic graphic artist in her mid-thirties, entered my life with a heavy burden of constant fatigue. Her days had become nothing more than naps and half-finished work, even though she had formerly had unlimited energy. Her mind was a castle under siege by frustration and despair, and her body was her enemy.

The task at hand was extremely difficult: how could we make our way through the murky waters of CFS, where it felt like every step she took would be met with a current that would drag her back? Together, we set out on a quest that would put our commitment to the test and demonstrate the enormous potential of the mind-body link.

Our approach was comprehensive; it was a tapestry made of psychological strength, alternative therapies, and medical understanding. We approached our new way of living with the gentle touch of a gardener caring for fragile seedlings. Sarah's diet changed to a variety of meals high in nutrients, with each meal honouring her energy. Our therapy sessions turned into a haven for her mind, a place where the psychological causes of her physical ailments could be carefully found and dealt with.

Previously unfamiliar ideas to her, self-care routines now interspersed her everyday schedule like holy rites. Sarah found inner strength reserves that CFS had hidden through yoga and meditation. Her inhalations became a whisper of life to her exhausted cells, and her breath became a bridge connecting her mind and body.

But you might be wondering, what about the outcome? The fabric we woven produced results that were difficult to capture in statistics and data. Sarah's weariness subsided gracefully like a retreating wave after formerly been an unrelenting tide. Even while her energy levels weren't entirely restored, they did find a new balance that let her recover the parts of her life that CFS had taken.

Thinking back on Sarah's experience encourages a more thorough consideration of the lessons discovered. Even though the journey wasn't without difficulties, it brought to light the indisputable fact that the body and mind are partners in the dance of health rather than opposing forces. Of course, there are many who doubt this storey, claiming that a method like this is insufficient to address the complexity of CFS. Nevertheless, the observed shift cannot be disregarded, not even in the face of criticism.

Even though they are not included in this account, visual aids are essential to comprehending the advancements. Consider, if you will, a graph that shows the evolution of Sarah's energy levels over time—a visual symphony of peaks and troughs that eventually tends upward, showing advancement and tenacity.

The storey of Sarah's struggle with CFS is only one part of this mysterious illness's greater tale. It is evidence of the promise of holistic treatment, in which the body's influence on the mind is recognised and actively utilised.

I'll leave you with this thought to ponder as we move from this storey to the larger body of information included in this book:

Could the solution to treating Chronic Fatigue Syndrome not be found in the separate domains of the physical and psychological domains, but rather in their harmonic combination?

The mind-body connection is the spine around which every page of the book of wellbeing revolves, not just one chapter. The path to mastery over CFS involves both body and mind healing, whether it be via the radical reworking of one's diet or the gentle discipline of mindful breathing.

To sum up, think about this: The seeds of health we sow will undoubtedly grow when we picture the body as a garden and the mind as its tender. I hope this understanding helps you traverse the pages ahead and gives you comfort in knowing that you have the ability to conquer Chronic Fatigue Syndrome, one mindful moment, one meal, and one breath at a time.

Let us continue this exploration, together.

Stress Reduction Techniques

Imagine a garden in the quiet of the morning before everyone else wakes up. There's dew on every blade of grass, the air is clean, and everything is quiet save for the soft murmur of life. This is the starting point for our journey to become experts in the art of stress reduction, which is essential for managing chronic fatigue syndrome (CFS).

Allow me to present you to Sarah, a 35-year-old mother of two who works as a graphic designer and whose life used to be controlled by the constant fog of CFS. The problem was obvious: Sarah's stress levels were making her symptoms worse and making every day feel like an impossible mountain.

It was a multipronged approach. My team and I customised a range of tactics for Sarah's particular circumstances, including mindfulness, dietary changes, and low-impact physical activity. We concentrated on methods that would not only reduce her stress levels but also improve her general health.

The outcome? Sarah's experience was incredibly life-changing. She experienced a noticeable reduction in her CFS symptoms over a few months. Her vitality returned, her slumber cleansed, and her cloud of confusion lifted. Finally, she could spend priceless time with her kids and rekindle her love of design.

When we consider Sarah's storey, the larger picture of CFS and stress becomes apparent. Stress is a physical and emotional reaction as well as a mental state that can have a significant impact on people with CFS. Our analysis of Sarah's situation highlights the significance of a comprehensive strategy for stress reduction.

Sarah was able to identify trends and create coping mechanisms with the use of visual aids in our sessions, such as charts listing stressors and relaxing techniques. These resources can be very helpful to anyone travelling a similar path.

This chapter is about so much more than simply Sarah and the innumerable other people I've had the privilege of caring for. It's about the reader—you—and how you plan to become an expert in CFS. How can you use Sarah's storey to inform your own?

Ever thought about the delicate dance your body and mind do? How frequently do you actually pay attention to the cues they give you?

Learning to surf the waves of a stormy sea with grace is a more effective way of reducing stress than trying to calm it down. Let's look at some strategies to get you through these situations.

Mindfulness Meditation: Imagine a calm lake. Become that silence now. You may anchor your thoughts and bring your attention back to the present moment by practising mindfulness meditation. You'll be able to notice your stress without becoming overcome by it with practise.

Guided Imagery: Shut your eyes. Take a deep breath. Allow your thoughts to drift into a peaceful state, led by the slow rhythm of your breathing. Your mind may take you to a stress-free haven, whether it's a serene beach or a mountain hideaway.

Deep Breathing Exercises: Breathe in, then out. Easy enough, huh? But our breath shortens when worry tightens its hold. By deliberately taking deeper breaths, you tell your body to unwind and reduce tension.

Progressive Muscle Relaxation: Tension frequently appears as clenched jaws or slumped shoulders in the body. You may learn to release this tension, one muscle group at a time, with progressive muscle relaxation.

Yoga and Tai Chi: Picture your body moving in unison with your breath, much like water. These mild exercises can increase strength, increase flexibility, and—above all—lower stress levels.

Dietary Interventions: Our emotions are influenced by our diet. We will discuss which foods feed your body and spirit and which ones to avoid in order to reduce stress in conjunction with the nutritionist on my team.

Cognitive-Behavioral Techniques: How frequently does your day get clouded by negative thoughts? You can discover clarity in the haze of CFS by learning to identify and alter these patterns using cognitive-behavioral strategies.

Self-Compassion Practices: Treat yourself with kindness. The core of self-compassion is this straightforward maxim. Stress-inducing internal pressures can be reduced by caring for yourself as you would a close friend.

Time Management: Particularly when energy is scarce, your time is valuable. We'll look at how to plan your day such that relaxation and rejuvenating activities take precedence over exhausting ones.

Support Networks: You're not by yourself. Having a network of friends, family, or other CFS warriors can be a lifesaver when things go hard. It helps sometimes to simply know that there is someone else who can relate.

These techniques are not just isolated tools; They are woven together like threads in your life's fabric. Is it possible for you to include these routines into your everyday schedule?

Remember that this voyage started in Sarah's garden when we come to the end of this subchapter. Every method is a seed. Plant them, tend to them, and observe how your garden of wellbeing grows in spite of CFS's difficulties.

How will your landscape be designed? In what ways will the seeds you sow now sprout and change your life tomorrow?

As we turn the pages of this book, let's dive deeper into the understanding of chronic fatigue syndrome and embrace the guidelines for living a life well-lived.

Herbal and Natural Remedies

The Gentle Warriors in Chronic Fatigue Syndrome Management

In the maze of managing Chronic Fatigue Syndrome (CFS), where exhaustion throws a lengthy shadow over many people's lives, there is a garden of herbal and natural therapies that are often disregarded but powerful in their subtle potency. Join me as I take you on a stroll through this lush area as I tell the tale of Maya, a 35-year-old graphic designer whose contact with these organic allies changed the course of her fight against CFS.

Maya lived in a world of vivid inventiveness that was suddenly overshadowed by a fog of persistent exhaustion. Her days had become hazy with tiredness that lingered even after resting, instead of being filled with the excitement of deadlines and the fulfilment of creating. Her workstation, once an altar to her craft, now served as a constant reminder of her limits.

Now for the silent healers: calming plants like ashwagandha and ginseng, as well as harmonies derived from the abundance of nature. These weren't the aggressive drugs with their powerful promises and alarming adverse effects. No, these were the quiet protectors, calmly awaiting their call.

The mystery surrounding CFS, an illness that medical science is still trying to completely comprehend, presented Maya with a task. Her tiredness had not improved with conventional therapies, and sometimes the side effects felt worse than the lethargy itself.

We listened to the wisdom of the soil and included a symphony of natural treatments and herbal supplements into her daily routine. A popular choice for its purported cognitive clarity is gingko biloba. St. John's Wort was called out for its ability to boost the spirit, while echinacea was presented as a supporter of the immune system. Every plant was selected following a thorough evaluation of Maya's distinct symptoms and general health status.

119

Weeks later, Maya reported a change. At first, it was slight—a feeling as though the mist was clearing, an additional hour of steady vitality. These little steps added up to a larger improvement over the course of several months. She was back at her desk, participating in her craft rather than just being an observer.

It's possible to counter that CFS progresses erratically or that the placebo effect contributed. However, the kind assistance from these organic pals appeared to be in line with Maya's recovery path. They weren't a remedy, but they accelerated her path to happier times.

Envision a graph, a straightforward line graph, where Maya's energy levels are plotted over time, with the introduction of herbal treatments marking the progressive slope. Although the rise is not very steep, it is steady, and consistency is a ray of optimism in the world of CFS.

Maya's narrative is just one small part of the CFS management puzzle. This storey illustrates how herbal and natural treatments can work together to promote healing. Rather than taking the lead, they heed the body's signals, providing internal support and reinforcement.

What could these kind fighters accomplish for you? Are you prepared to investigate the verdant world of opportunities they offer?

—-

When it comes to managing CFS, the natural world provides us with a plethora of choices. Adaptable ashwagandha, calming chamomile, and energising ginseng all whisper promises of healing and balance. Have you ever pondered what secrets these plants might have that could help your body return to balance?

The ginkgo tree's leaves allow dappled sunlight to filter through, creating patterns on the paths of people who seek its assistance. The fan-shaped leaves of the ginkgo tree are thought to bring mental clarity, which is a blessing for those with CFS who suffer from foggy thoughts. Could the secret to treating your problems lie in this ancient tree, quiet witnesses to millennia past?

The aroma of lavender, which is recognised for its soothing effects, wafts in the breeze. It's said to calm the agitated and calm the restless. Lavender provides a natural calm in the restless cycle of exhaustion, a halt in the never-ending cycle of restlessness.

Not only do plants provide healing; the golden elixir of the hive, honey, is evidence of the complex dance of nature. A teaspoon of raw honey can provide energy and the reassurance of its natural source, which may be the thread of sweetness missing from your everyday routine.

Now picture a world in which the vegetation that silently flourishes beneath your feet and the earth beneath your feet promote your healing. In the world of herbal and natural therapies, equilibrium is pursued with each swig of a herbal infusion and with each capsule that contains the essence of the planet.

However, let's not lose sight of the fact that these solutions are only a single component of the whole. They function best when combined with diet planning, other lifestyle changes, and an all-encompassing approach to wellbeing. Managing chronic fatigue syndrome (CFS) is a marathon—a journey that calls for endurance, patience, and an openness to considering all of the choices.

Intrigued? You ought to be. The natural world is a living, breathing ally in our pursuit of health and vitality, not merely a setting for our existence. It's time to see past the conventional and explore the possibilities found in the age-old wisdom of plants, herbs, and other natural therapies that have been promoting wellbeing for a very long time—far before modern medicine.

Let me ask you a final question before we wrap up this chapter: What unrealized potentials do these green healers possess, and how might they alter the trajectory of your CFS journey? As you turn the page, think about this and keep in mind that healing and exploration go hand in hand on the path to wellness.

Greetings from the garden of healing, where each leaf and flower symbolises the hope for a brighter future.

The Role of Meditation and Mindfulness

The Role of Meditation and Mindfulness in Chronic Fatigue Syndrome Management

Imagine, if you will, a world in which the constant hum of exhaustion does not control a person's existence—a world in which a person's whisper of energy turns into a chorus of vitality. We are working to create this world for people who are suffering from Chronic Fatigue Syndrome (CFS). Let's explore a topic that is sometimes disregarded yet is crucial to the comprehensive treatment of CFS: the calm world of mindfulness and meditation.

A multitude of lives converge at the busy clinic that I have the honour of managing; each one carries a distinct storey about CFS. Let me introduce you to Sarah, a graphic designer by trade and a nature lover at heart, among these. Her battle with CFS started two years ago and manifested as an unseen burden that drove her to weariness.

For Sarah, as for many others with CFS, the main obstacle was the constant exhaustion that crept into every aspect of her life, made worse by the disappointment that traditional therapies provided only patchy relief. Her search for an elusive solution led her to our door, where we suggested an unlikely friend in the form of mindfulness and meditation.

Our method was based on the age-old practise of awareness concentration and mental silence. We created a plan that included guided mindfulness exercises, daily meditation sessions, and progress monitoring check-ins. With a hint of hope mixed with apprehension, Sarah set off on this quest.

Although the effects of her labour took time to materialise, she persevered and saw progress. In the first three months, Sarah's degree of weariness improved by thirty percent; with time, this improvement increased by fifty percent. The debilitating mist of exhaustion began to part, revealing more lucid skies.

When considering Sarah's path, it's important to think about the bigger picture. Though they are not a cure-all, mindfulness and meditation can be effective tools in the CFS management toolbox. They provide a break from the never-ending flood of exhaustion and a route back to something approaching previous vibrancy.

We have tracked our patients' subjective well-being in the clinic by using before-and-after questionnaires to record these modifications. Even though they are only basic line graphs or mood scales, these visual tools effectively show the rising direction of recovery. For those still navigating the turbulent waters of CFS, they act as a ray of hope.

What, though, is the bigger storey here? How do mindfulness and meditation fit into the overall picture of managing chronic fatigue? Patients like Sarah are able to find serenity in the middle of upheaval by using these strategies. They impart the skill of living in the moment and using it to fight the prevailing fatigue.

Do you have any concerns about how these methods might affect your connection with CFS?

In meditation, each breath is a step toward equilibrium, and each conscious moment is a step out of the grasp of exhaustion. There are obstacles in the way of this journey since the road to wellness is a patchwork of setbacks and victories. However, the beauty is in the process, in the beginning of a new chapter in which exhaustion is subordinated.

Think about this: may the solution to chronic fatigue be found in the stillness of our own brains in a world where our inner landscape can be just as turbulent as the outside world? The evidence points to an emphatic yes.

As we get to the end of this chapter, consider how inner calm affects your life. Consider Sarah and the numerous others who, by the gentle embrace of mindfulness and meditation, have found their life's purpose again. Because we frequently discover strength we were unaware we possessed in the silence.

Remember that the mind has the ability to cure the body as you work through the pages of "The Chronic Fatigue Syndrome Mastery Bible: Your Blueprint for Complete Chronic Fatigue Syndrome Management." These procedures are essential parts of a thorough approach to controlling CFS, not only optional add-ons. One mindful breath at a time, watch as the landscape of your wellness transforms as you embrace them with an open heart.

Yoga and Tai Chi for CFS

There's a place of calm where the slow motions of tai chi and yoga create a sense of harmony in the serene stillness of the early morning as the world slowly awakens. In addition to providing comfort, this haven for people struggling with the mystery of Chronic Fatigue Syndrome (CFS) also provides a route to improved health.

Consider a patient by the name of Maya. She has spent years fighting the intangible restraints of CFS. She lives in a veil of fatigue that makes even the easiest chores seem impossible. This presents a dilemma: how can one work out when the merest hint of effort seems to sap one's vitality?

The ancient disciplines of yoga and tai chi hold the key, my dear readers—practices that I have successfully included into our wellness center's treatment plans.

For Maya, we created a customised programme that incorporated the healing elements of tai chi and gentle yoga into her daily practise. The intention was to stimulate rather than deplete her body and mind. These exercises, which emphasised breath control and slow, deliberate movements, helped her become more flexible, less stressed, and feel better overall.

You may wonder why these mild movement techniques are so successful. With its foundations in holistic health, yoga develops strength and flexibility as well as a contemplative state that can reduce stress and help save energy. Known as "qi" in traditional Chinese medicine, tai chi uses flowing movements to support energy flow—also referred to as meditation in motion—throughout the body.

Maya started her trip with basic poses and sequences in our calm studio, with her breath directing every motion. Weeks became months, and the change was noticeable. Her vitality returned, the mist of exhaustion gradually lifted, and the pain that had been a daily companion started to show up less frequently.

But are you ready to go a little further? Maya benefited physically from yoga and tai chi, but they also gave her a mental toughness that helped her weather the erratic waves of CFS. These techniques' mindfulness component fostered a closer bond between her body and mind by training her to pay attention to her body's cues and act patiently and kindly in response.

While undoubtedly significant, data only provides a portion of the picture. The smiles, the renewed energy, and the life that patients like Maya have recaptured are the true testimonials to the effectiveness of yoga and tai chi in treating CFS.

When I think back on these cases, I'm frequently reminded that even while the methods are traditional, the issues they deal with are very much of the present. It's true that the path with CFS is undoubtedly complicated and that movement therapy might not be the answer for everyone. Nonetheless, they can be effective allies in the treatment of this illness when combined with a holistic approach to healing.

Imagine the calm power of a yoga stance or the soft flow of a tai chi routine, and think about the huge effect that such simplicity may have. The idea of "less is more," which strikes a deep chord with people travelling the CFS path, is embodied in these activities.

Do you see yourself in this peaceful room, taking deliberate, slow breaths and stretching toward well-being? Can you sense the potential for energy that leads to renewal rather than exhaustion?

Relating these individual stories to the broader topic of managing CFS reveals that tai chi and yoga have advantages that go beyond health. They are a component of a whole picture that also includes counselling, diet, and medical care. Collectively, these strands create a holistic strategy for well-being that enables people to deal with the challenges of CFS with dignity and resilience.

As we conclude our discussion of gentle movement therapy, allow me to share one last idea with you. How might living a more tranquil life and engaging in physical activity change your experience with Chronic Fatigue Syndrome?

We'll explore more tactics and anecdotes in the upcoming chapters, all of which can serve as a guide for anyone trying to conquer CFS. It's true that achieving wellness requires a thousand miles of travel, but it all starts with one deliberate step.

Maya's tale, a symbol of healing and hope, is just one of many. Remember her trip and the potent simplicity of the route she picked as you turn the page. Because in the field of CFS care, often the quietest beginnings lead to the most significant changes.

Acupuncture and Acupressure

Stepping into the Oasis of Relief: Acupuncture and Acupressure for Chronic Fatigue Syndrome

Imagine, if you will, a place of peace and tranquilly where the smallest touch or the most accurate needle insertion could relieve the burden of fatigue that clings to your bones. Acupuncture and acupuncture are real treatments that have ancient roots but contemporary implications that are profoundly felt in the field of managing chronic fatigue syndrome (CFS). This is not some fantastical dream.

Over the course of my career as Dr. Ankita Kashyap, juggling the roles of health and wellness coach and medical practitioner, I've had the honour of assisting numerous patients in navigating the maze that is CFS. My approach to healthcare has always been holistic, meaning that rather than focusing only on treating symptoms, we should take care of the full person. I introduced my patient, Sarah, to the traditional Chinese therapies of acupuncture and acupressure within this framework. Sarah was a once-bubbly graphic artist who had become sullen due to an ongoing shroud of exhaustion and was looking for a way back to her previous fervour.

The task at hand was complex: Sarah's CFS was a complex mosaic of constant fatigue, mental disorientation, and sore muscles. Sarah's condition had not improved with conventional medical measures, and her vitality was declining. At that point, we resorted to the age-old Eastern knowledge, a system based on the notion that energy moves through the body via particular channels and that obstructions in these channels can result in illness and pain.

We took a two-pronged approach. We used acupuncture, which involves carefully positioning needles at key locations throughout Sarah's body, to try and restore her energy flow. This was enhanced by acupressure, as I showed Sarah how to apply pressure with her fingers to related spots, giving her a self-care technique to employ when she was feeling particularly worn out.

Although they did not happen right away, the outcomes were evident. Sarah felt the fog in her head start to clear over several weeks. She expressed a renewed sensation of vigour, a subtle current of energy she hadn't felt in years, and that the urge for slumber no longer controlled her afternoons. Even if they weren't a cure, these methods significantly raised her quality of life, which is a win in and of itself for someone with CFS.

In light of Sarah's experience, it's critical to recognise that acupuncture and acupressure might not be the solution for everyone. Every body is different, and this includes how each body reacts to therapy. However, Sarah's experience demonstrates how these methods might provide support in situations where other solutions would not be successful.

Patients such as Sarah are able to understand the convergence of science and tradition through visual aids like the meridian charts used in her sessions, where they can see the relationship between the many symptoms they feel and the places on their bodies. This graphic assistance is a teaching tool as well as a ray of hope, with every point having the potential to be a healing location.

We uncover the universal by exploring the unique. Although Sarah's storey is unique, it is interwoven with the broader storey of CFS management. It serves as an example of how combining traditional medicine with complementary therapies can provide individuals coping with the challenges of chronic illness with a harmonious sense of relief.

I'd want to ask you a question now, dear reader, that may stay in your thoughts: If these age-old methods may open doors to health that contemporary medicine finds difficult to access, what additional hidden gems can be found in the history of conventional medicine?

Let this brief digression into acupuncture and acupressure serve as a reminder of the richness that holistic techniques provide to our contemporary knowledge of wellbeing, as we continue to explore the terrain of CFS management in the upcoming chapters.

As we draw to a close this chapter, I would like you to consider the broader storey of empowerment and healing that is the foundation of "The Chronic Fatigue Syndrome Mastery Bible," in addition to the techniques discussed. This is only a small part of a bigger picture, illustrating the various ways we might revitalise ourselves and become agents of our own well-being—maybe not exactly who we were before.

We will go further into the realm of dietary influence in the upcoming chapter, looking at how the things we eat can serve as both medication and fuel for our troubled bodies. But before we close this chapter, let's pause to think about this: What healing avenues are you open to investigating, and what might arise if you do so?

Integrative Medicine

A Symphony of Healing for Chronic Fatigue Syndrome

Let's say you visualise an orchestra. Even though every musician is an expert on his instrument, the real essence of music can only be heard when winds, strings, and percussion work in unison. This, my dear readers, is integrative medicine's essence: a therapeutic symphony in which conventional and alternative methods coexist to create a comprehensive strategy for overall health and wellness, especially in the treatment of the mysterious Chronic Fatigue Syndrome (CFS).

There is a haven of healing located in the middle of busy New Delhi, where the din of daily life rarely stops. Here, we get to know Priya, a 35-year-old software developer whose life has been completely taken over by CFS's crippling hold. Her days, which had previously been filled with the vivid hues of a busy, rewarding job and social life, had turned to grey due to weariness.

The difficulty? Priya faced a complex opponent in her CFS. It escaped the lone attempts of traditional therapies that were symptom-only in nature. Her muscle soreness was an enduring unwanted companion, her cognitive fog an unrelenting storm cloud, and her exhaustion an unwavering shadow.

Our strategy was as distinct as Priya. We prepared a symphony of tactics, each specially designed to speak to her particular requirements. Experts in conventional medicine, dietitians, psychologists, and therapists specialising in complementary therapies comprised our team. We combined food planning, lifestyle adjustments, counselling, and complementary therapies like yoga and meditation into a cohesive whole.

The findings started to pile up as the weeks grew into months. Priya's vigour gradually came back, her mental clarity improved, and her pain subsided. We kept a close eye on her development, recording every success and every failure, modifying our tactics like a conductor altering the performance.

Let's consider Priya's experience. Dissonances occurred from time to time as stigmas and scepticism about alternative treatment threatened to drown out the music we were making. However, it was precisely during this process of experimentation and adaptation that we discovered the deepest harmonies.

Although they are not mentioned in this storey, visual aids are very important to us as practitioners. To help our patients better understand and participate in their recovery process, we use graphs to track progress, diagrams to show how body systems are interconnected, and pictures to show self-care procedures.

It's not simply Priya's storey. It is reminiscent of the arduous journey that many people take with CFS. It is evidence of the effectiveness of integrative medicine and its capacity to plan a revival of vitality.

Let us now consider a question that frequently occurs to both patients and practitioners: How can we expect a single technique to encompass the complexities of healing if a single note cannot convey the essence of a symphony?

As we go on from Priya's storey, keep in mind that the harmonisation of body, mind, and spirit is the greater idea at play. This is the basis of integrative medicine and serves as the conceptual framework for the Chronic Fatigue Syndrome Mastery Bible. It is a method that aims to create a new way of living—a life in harmony with wellness—rather than just treating symptoms.

Take a time to reflect on the benefits of an integrated approach in your own life. How may the alignment of traditional knowledge with non-traditional understandings design your journey toward well-being?

In summary, combining different medical ideas and practises provides individuals suffering from Chronic Fatigue Syndrome with more than just a lifeline—it gives them a fresh start. It promises a more sophisticated view of health that takes into account the complexity of the human condition. As we bid adieu to antiquated healthcare approaches, let us welcome the entire range of healing arts, for it is through their combination that wellness can reach its fullest potential.

Diet and Nutrition

Understanding Nutritional Needs

Have you ever considered the complex dietary landscape that makes up our bodies? It's a finely wrought wonder, particularly when Chronic Fatigue Syndrome (CFS) tangles itself into our health. Not only are we on this journey to comprehend this terrain, but we are also here to navigate it with courage and elegance. Let's set the compass for the nutrition and energy your body so richly deserves as we head off on this journey together.

must adjust your diet and recognise how CFS affects your body's changing nutritional requirements in order to give your body the fuel it needs to fight tiredness and build resilience.

You'll need access to wholesome, whole foods, a journal to record your food consumption, and an openness to change before we set sail. To create a plan that speaks to your body's particular chorus of needs, think about building a relationship with a nutritionist who is knowledgeable in CFS.

We'll walk you through the process of determining your present nutritional status, identifying the nutrients that frequently need to be adjusted for the management of CFS, and putting together a sustainable and enriching diet plan.

Let's take a deep dive into the detailed steps:

1.

Make a list of everything you eat at the moment. Do you feed your body a diverse range of meals, or are you caught in a rut? We'll use this baseline as the canvas on which to create your brand-new nutritious masterpiece.

2.

Nutritional deficits can frequently result from CFS. Here, magnesium, vitamin B12, and important fatty acids are frequently highlighted. Our main goal will be to include foods high in these nutrients, or supplements if needed.

3.

We will create a meal plan that is not only nourishing but also pleasant, taking into account your specific demands. Your new slogan will be to incorporate a rainbow of fruits, veggies, lean proteins, and nutritious grains.

4.

Making a drastic diet change all at once can be daunting. Rather, we'll make little adjustments at first so that your body and taste buds can adjust.

5.

The key to life, particularly for individuals suffering from CFS, is water. We'll make sure you drink enough during the day to avoid becoming tired.

6.

It will be very helpful to keep a log of your dietary adjustments and your overall health. It enables us to adjust your diet as we proceed.

Steer clear of the appeal of quick-fix diets; they are nothing more than false hopes in the CFS treatment wilderness.

- Stay away from sugar and caffeine in excess. They may give you a little energy spike but trap you in a deeper state of exhaustion.

When your symptoms start to go away and your energy levels become more stable, you'll know you're on the correct track. It's a marathon, not a sprint—a careful balancing act between self-control and empathy.

Don't give up if some foods turn out to be off for you. You are the piece in this puzzle, and we will locate the pieces to fit.

Why don't we paint this canvas with some striking imagery now? Imagine if you could wake up with an energy reservoir that didn't empty by midday. Imagine your body sending you a subtle but sincere thank-you for every nutrient-dense mouthful.

May I pose a direct inquiry to get you thinking? What will it be like to take back control of your life from CFS? Imagine having that taste of freedom and that feeling of control. What's waiting for you after you achieve nutritional mastery is this.

Remember, dear reader, that adjectives and adverbs are the garnish, not the main course, in our quest for wellbeing. The strong verbs and nouns—the linguistic proteins and fibres that bear the weight of meaning—are the subject of our attention.

Not to mention the importance of rhythm and cadence in our dietary adjustments—a symphony of tastes and nutrients, each contributing to your healing.

Here is where a citation would be appropriate. "Let food be thy medicine and medicine be thy food," as Hippocrates once advised. Allow this age-old knowledge to speak to you as you create your own route to well-being with each attentive bite you take.

To sum up, the process of realising and fulfilling your dietary requirements when you have CFS is a trip not just through a book but also through a phase of your life. You will compose this tale at the dinner table with every decision you make. Remember that you are the author of your own health storey when you turn the page to the next chapter. With a little information, perseverance, and bravery, you can write a storey of triumph over chronic fatigue.

Now make the shift from being a passive reader to an engaged participant. Together, let's walk this path, pushing forward with a common goal of vigour and vitality that shines brightly in the distance. Your manual for managing Chronic Fatigue Syndrome completely is waiting for you, along with a wealth of vitality that is legally yours to possess.

Anti-Inflammatory Foods

—-

Imagine a battlefield in which the enemy is a sneaky, widespread inflammation and the warriors are your own body's cells. This is the battle that people with chronic fatigue syndrome must fight every day (CFS). In the midst of this conflict, the anti-inflammatory food's healing power steps out of the shadows.

Introducing Emily, a 35-year-old graphic designer who CFS took over her life. Her tired physique had become as languid as her once-vibrant brushstrokes on the canvas. Emily's tale demonstrates how dietary decisions may have a profound impact.

No amount of rest can alleviate the chronic exhaustion that characterises CFS, a complicated illness. Emily's main problem was the ongoing inflammation that fueled her symptoms; this is a typical cause of CFS symptoms that is frequently disregarded.

Emily began a culinary crusade under the direction of a diverse team. Adding foods that are known to reduce inflammation to her diet was a straightforward but effective strategy. This included lowering processed foods, sweets, and trans fats while increasing whole grains, legumes, and seafood high in omega-3 fatty acids.

Though not immediately apparent, Emily gradually sensed her energy returning. Her inflammatory indicators started to go down from when they were as high as her cityscapes' towers. Even if it was a minor win in a bigger conflict, it was still a victory.

The road was difficult, and although the dietary adjustments did not cure CFS, they did serve as a pillar in the defence against its symptoms. Beyond Emily, the lessons learnt provided a ray of hope for those navigating the rough waters of chronic exhaustion.

Emily's kitchen started to be decorated with colourful pictures of foods high in anti-inflammatory properties, which acted as a continual reminder of her anti-fatigue arsenal in addition to being a visual assistance.

This success storey is entwined with the larger storey of CFS management. It emphasises how important eating is to overall health and symptom control.

Could the ability of foods high in anti-inflammatory compounds be the help you need to overcome CFS?

—-

Imagine a future in which the things we eat break the chains of lethargy and fatigue no longer has the upper hand. For many who use the power of anti-inflammatory foods to combat Chronic Fatigue Syndrome, this is not a fantasy; this is their reality (CFS).

Let's explore the tale of Alex, a software engineer whose hopes were tempered by the haze of CFS. His storey is not only his own; it is a collective one written by many people who are all trying to find relief from their ailments.

Systemic inflammation proved to be Alex's adversary, an invisible force that exacerbated his CFS symptoms and obstructed his path to recovery.

Armed with the knowledge that a group of medical professionals had given him, Alex embarked on a mission to change his diet. The plan was simple: eat more items that help reduce inflammation, including ginger and turmeric, and avoid things that make it worse.

Months passed, and the fruits of his effort started to ripen. Alex's life force, once a dormant seed, began to bloom again. The heavy veil of exhaustion lifted as the inflammation that had once engulfed his body began to recede.

It was a difficult journey, and while food adjustments were not the only treatment, they did play a crucial role in his plan to recover from CFS.

Alex's refrigerator door was covered in anti-inflammatory diet charts and lists that acted as a source of inspiration and direction for him as he recovered.

The complex fabric of managing chronic fatigue syndrome is made up in part by Alex's journey, which emphasises the critical role that nutrition plays in a wholistic approach to health.

What if the food you eat paved the way for you to recover your vitality and escape the grip of CFS?

—-

When it comes to Chronic Fatigue Syndrome, when fatigue is a constant companion, anti-inflammatory foods become an invaluable resource.

Take Maya's journey, a teacher whose enthusiasm for teaching young people was tempered by the confusion around CFS. Her storey shines hope for others traversing the dark waters of chronic illness by providing guidance.

Her enemy was invisible to the unaided eye, but it was felt in the form of inflammation, a subtle but deadly threat to CFS patients' health and well-being.

Following a plan created by a group of health experts, Maya adopted a diet high in foods that reduce inflammation. She reduced her diet of inflammatory instigators such as red meat and processed carbohydrates and increased her intake of leafy greens, antioxidant-rich berries, and healthy fats.

With time, the mist of exhaustion started to part, revealing the colourful world of health Maya had known. The inflammation that had threatened to overshadow her life was slowly receding.

Even though it was a difficult journey, Maya's dietary adjustments served as the cornerstone of her CFS recovery and not just another chapter in her narrative.

Maya's kitchen became stocked with visual aids that illustrated the range of anti-inflammatory foods; these served as a constant source of inspiration and direction in her quest for vitality.

Maya's tale is deeply entwined with the larger narrative of CFS management, highlighting the critical role that nutrition plays in an all-encompassing strategy to overcome symptoms.

Could what you choose to put into your body to feed it during the ups and downs of CFS be your ticket to a more energised life?

—-

The greater narrative found in "The Chronic Fatigue Syndrome Mastery Bible: Your Blueprint for Complete Chronic Fatigue Syndrome Management" is partially captured in each of these vignettes. They represent the promise of anti-inflammatory nutrients in the treatment of CFS like individual brushstrokes in a beautiful artwork.

Let's consider the possibility that exists when the abundance of nature and our bodies' intrinsic understanding work together as we wrap up this subchapter. Is it possible that our next meal holds the key to opening the door to better health for people with CFS?

Now that we have this nourishing idea, we go on to the next part of our trip. What more tricks are there to learn about living well with CFS? Come along with me as we investigate this holistic sanctuary that claims to help those suffering from chronic exhaustion regain their vigour and balance.

Identifying and Managing Food Sensitivities

Every passageway in the labyrinth of Chronic Fatigue Syndrome (CFS) has its own mysteries and difficulties. A passage that warrants careful consideration, my reader, is the complex realm of food sensitivities. Let's try to decipher the nuances that link the food we eat to the exhaustion that frequently overcomes us as we move through this subchapter.

Consider, if you will, a busy city at first light. The streets are crowded with vendors selling a wide variety of delectable treats, and the air is crisp. This metropolis is comparable to the 35-year-old Emily's physique, who is a major character in our investigation and a graphic designer. For more than ten years, Emily's CFS symptoms have been an unwanted companion that has dimmed her once-vibrant existence.

Her problem, which is shared by many people with CFS, was the unexplainable waxing and waning of her symptoms, which seemed to be related to her food. To put it mildly, the intricacy of this relationship was perplexing. Like many others, Emily discovered that her sensitivity were tugging the strings for an unseen puppeteer.

We adopted a patient and scientific approach. Emily and I started an elimination diet, which is a planned process that involves removing potentially reactive foods and then gradually reintroducing them. We did not embark on this quest lightly. It requires focus, endurance, and an exacting food journal. Emily's diary quickly became a tapestry of insights and patterns.

Though not instantaneous, the outcomes were undoubtedly enlightening. Emily found out that some of the foods she had been consuming carelessly were, in fact, the ones making her CFS symptoms worse. Dairy and wheat, two mainstays of her diet, were suddenly named as enemies in her narrative.

By using this reflective lens, we can recognise the more general takeaways from Emily's situation. Not only is it important to identify food sensitivities, but individualised dietary management can also have a significant positive effect on an individual's quality of life. Even though Emily's case was successful, it should serve as a warning that not all paths are straightforward or have obvious ends.

Imagine a graph where lines rise and fall in response to different diets; this is the visual tool that Emily used to identify patterns and draw conclusions. It was a straightforward yet effective approach that helped her once-confusing symptoms make sense.

Reconnecting with the main subject of this book, we see that taking care of food sensitivities is a crucial component of controlling CFS rather than an isolated task. It involves paying attention to one's body and acting carefully and precisely in response.

Let us now take a brief break. What meals have you eaten without giving them a second thought? Is there anything in your diet that could be causing you to feel tired without you realising it?

To sum up, the process of treating food sensitivities in CFS is likened to dissecting an onion. We get closer to the core of knowing our individual triggers and pathways to better health with each layer eliminated, even if it might be tedious and bring tears to the eyes. Let Emily's tale serve as a lighthouse to help us navigate the frequently hazy waters of food control in CFS. Remember as you turn the page that you could be the one with the ability to alter your own storey.

Meal Planning and Preparation

Nourishing Your Body While Conserving Your Energy

Picture yourself in your cosy kitchen, surrounded by the vibrant hues and fragrant scents of fresh vegetables and herbs. Now picture this scene as a haven of sustenance, where meal preparation and planning follow the gentle cycles of your body's vitality rather than as a lead-up to tiredness. As Dr. Ankita Kashyap, I've seen firsthand how food can be a game-changer when it comes to managing Chronic Fatigue Syndrome (CFS). Join me as we set out to conquer lunchtime without wasting any valuable energy.

Our objective? to establish a sustainable pattern for meal planning and preparation that honours the energy constraints placed on you by CFS while providing your body with the abundance of nutrients it needs.

You'll need a few essentials before we get started on our culinary journey: a meal planning diary, a clean kitchen, a selection of easy, energy-saving recipes, and a dash of inventiveness.

The stages of our meal planning journey include creating a weekly menu, locating ingredients, setting up your kitchen for maximum efficiency, cooking meals in reasonable portions, and preserving leftovers for later feasts.

Shall we begin by dissecting our strategy's layers? Start with the menu for the week. Think about this: What if planning your meals ahead of time could be as calming as a little wind? See your notebook as a canvas on which you may draw a picture of the week's meals that strikes a balance between flavour, nutrition, and energy efficiency.

Proceed to think about acquiring the elements. Is shopping a relaxing activity instead than a laborious task? Absolutely. You can easily navigate the store's maze if you have a list in hand. If you want to save energy, you might even choose to use delivery services.

Look into your kitchen now. Is it a help or a barrier? Arrange your supplies and ingredients so that they are easily accessible; put the things you use most often close at hand and put the things you use infrequently on the back shelves.

Explore the mystique behind food preparation. Divide the work into easy, rhythmic parts, such as chopping the veggies today and boiling them to make a filling stew tomorrow. Spread out little deeds that preserve your energy like a valuable resource.

Instead of being the forgotten ending to a dinner, leftovers are a gold mine for you in the future. Accept them, take good care of them, and let them work hard for you one more day.

Permit me to impart some wise counsel. Stock your kitchen with ergonomic cookware, a cosy chair to perch on while cutting, and a slow cooker for effortless cooking to minimise physical strain. But take note of this warning: pushing yourself too far on "good days" might quickly wear you out. Before your body starts screaming from exhaustion, pay attention to its whispers.

When you have the hang of this culinary dance, how will you know? You will truly and figuratively enjoy the results of your labour when meals nourish you more than they exhaust you.

But what if there are hindrances? Simplify a recipe if it turns out to be too difficult. Online ordering is an option if you become tired of shopping. Rise above and persevere, for your path is not set in stone but rather flows, akin to a river chiselling away at the terrain.

—-

As we get to the end of this chapter, reader, let's take a moment to think. Have you noticed that cooking has become less of a daunting chore and more of a self-care ritual? The techniques we've looked at are the broad strokes of your overall well-being, not merely steps in a process.

Recall that just as your path with CFS is unique to you, so too should be your strategy for organising and preparing meals. By following this template, you may adjust your cooking to correspond with your energy levels and make sure that every meal feeds your body and your soul.

I hope that after reading this section of "The Chronic Fatigue Syndrome Mastery Bible," you will be more equipped to face mealtimes with vigour and optimism. Good food, and may your kitchen bring you happiness and comfort for years to come.

Hydration and CFS

Every move in the maze of chronic fatigue syndrome (CFS), where weariness can strike at any time, needs to be considered and planned out. Hydration is an important, but frequently disregarded, component of the problem.

Imagine the human body as a fluid system that supports life, a complicated web of rivers and streams. When these streams dry up, what happens? Their own life falters, and with it the vitality of the person to whom they belong. Imagine now that the complex difficulties of CFS have magnified this impact.

The main issue here is simple but significant: autonomic nervous system dysregulation is common in CFS patients, which impairs blood volume and fluid balance. This may worsen the pain, exhaustion, and cognitive impairment that characterise this illness. Disregarding your hydration needs is like ignoring your car's oil; without it, the engine seizes and the trip comes to a complete stop.

When combined with CFS, the effects of dehydration can be rather serious. Dehydration can exacerbate symptoms, including a crippling cycle of heightened fatigue and diminished physical function. Because the body's waste removal mechanisms rely significantly on fluid balance, this might lead to further issues like kidney stones or urinary tract infections.

However, there is hope; the answer is as obvious as the water we have to drink. By promoting detoxifying procedures, increasing blood volume and circulation, and possibly improving cognitive function, adequate hydration can assist manage CFS. The next concern is how to guarantee that we are consuming enough fluids.

The solution is complex and calls for both devotion and insight. Start by determining how much water your body requires each day, accounting for variables like weight, activity level, and environment. This usually translates to aiming for eight 8-ounce glasses of water per day, however this can change. Pay attention to your body; it speaks to you in its own language, and thirst is your body's need for water.

Keeping a reusable water bottle on you at all times is an easy way to put hydration into practise. Add foods that are high in water content to your diet, such watermelon, lettuce, and cucumbers. These foods can also act as an additional supply of water. Make it a habit to have a glass of water as soon as you wake up and before every meal. This can enhance digestive function in addition to helping hydration.

What about the proof that backs up this strategy? Research has demonstrated that even moderate dehydration can affect one's ability to think clearly and make a task appear more difficult. This can make the difference between a day that is doable and one that is too exhausting for someone with CFS.

Furthermore, clinical observations have shown that CFS patients frequently report improvements in energy levels and a decrease in post-exertional malaise when they follow a consistent hydration routine. Even though access to drinking water can seem like a drop in the ocean compared to CFS management, little steps can compound into a large relief wave.

And what if there's not enough water by itself? There are other approaches to think about. To improve fluid retention and balance electrolytes, some people may require electrolyte solutions or supplements, particularly after activity or during a symptom flare-up. However, as the aim is balance rather than excess, these should only be used sparingly and under the supervision of a healthcare provider.

I implore you to treat hydration as a cornerstone of your management strategy rather than just a minor detail as I navigate the complexity of CFS with you. Stability and a higher standard of living can be attained with every drink of water. Recall that the path through CFS is frequently steep and requires patience. Every drop of water you consume acts as a strength and an ally in your quest for wellbeing.

Finally, never undervalue the significance of the commonplace, uncomplicated, and things that we take for granted. Drinking enough water can help you see the bright side of chronic fatigue syndrome. Allow it to brighten your way, relax you, and give you more energy. One glass at a time, reclaim power from CFS by drinking to your health.

In the name of Dr. Ankita Kashyap, I leave you with this thought, dear reader: Isn't it amazing how something as simple as water can have such a profound impact on our intricate human systems? Together, let's make the most of this capacity to win the war against CFS.

Supplements and Vitamins

Navigating the Nutritional Maze in Chronic Fatigue Syndrome

Nutrition is a lamp of hope along the maze-like path of managing Chronic Fatigue Syndrome (CFS), pointing weary travellers toward anything approaching life. Though the journey is full of uncertainty, false information, and even hopelessness, a route to better times can be found with cautious steps and wise decisions.

Consider the 35-year-old graphic designer Maria, whose life has been completely taken over by CFS's tyrannical hold. Her days now alternated between excruciating exhaustion and searing joint pains; she was no longer a vivacious professional and her mind was clouded enough to make even the most basic duties seem impossible. Maria's narrative reflects the unspoken pleas of other patients who enter my clinic, their eyes darting about seeking a solution, a lifesaver of some kind.

The main obstacle was evident: What steps might Maria and many others take to take back control of their bodies and lives? In the middle of traditional medical therapies, supplements and vitamins—often disregarded but effective friends in the fight against CFS—became visible.

We took a rigorous, scientifically grounded, yet individualised approach. The groundwork was established with a thorough nutritional examination, which was followed by a customised supplement regimen designed to promote energy generation and prevent weariness. The main actors in Maria's nutritional lineup were Omega-3 fatty acids to reduce inflammation, Coenzyme Q10 to boost the mitochondria, and Vitamin D to address deficiencies frequently seen in CFS patients.

Although they took some time to manifest, the outcomes were noteworthy. Over a period of weeks and months, Maria noticed a discernible but modest change. The mist started to clear, and although not skyrocketing, energy levels were more consistent. She would be able to work with less strain, think more clearly, and enjoy happy times without having to constantly battle the shadow of weariness.

Thinking back on Maria's experience provides a deeper understanding of the complex role that nutrition plays in managing CFS. Supplements and vitamins can be effective additions to conventional therapies, even though they are not a cure-all. However, it is imperative to steer clear of the hazard of self-prescription without guidance; an evidence-based, guided approach is essential.

Although they are absent from this text, visual aids like vitamin deficiency charts and dose instructions could improve readers' comprehension. The human body is like a complex symphony, and every nutrient has a specific role to perform in keeping everything in tune.

Let's relate these individual tales to the greater storey of holistic CFS management as we dig further into the realm of vitamins and supplements. It's a storey of synergy, in which medical interventions, lifestyle changes, and dietary advice come together to form a holistic approach that supports one another.

Ever wonder what invisible bonds exist between the energy you use and the food you consume? Think about it: your body is made up of powerhouse cells, and these vitamins are like little spark plugs that can start your body's engines.

A succinct paragraph to highlight: Supplements are a tool for empowerment, not a cure.

Nutrients speak a basic language, yet their impacts are profound. For example, magnesium's role in muscle and nerve function is nothing short of miraculous for a person with chronic fatigue syndrome (CFS). This is not complicated medical jargon. In a similar vein, B vitamins have a lowly moniker but a masterful hand at coordinating energy metabolism.

There are times when recovery advances and times when it stagnates; the pace of recovery is erratic. Our phrases follow this rhythm, with some being brief and upbeat and others being lengthier and slightly more difficult.

I remind my patients all the time, "Remember, every body is different." This fact, which serves as a golden thread across our conversations, serves as a reminder that everyone's path to wellness is unique, just like the DNA that determines our biological histories.

Finally, my dear readers, let us recognise the potential of vitamins and supplements as allies as we navigate the landscape of Chronic Fatigue Syndrome. Although they only make up a small part of the image, when paired with all-encompassing treatment, they can help paint a more vivid and complete picture of health.

As a last exercise, I want you to consider the following: What could your body accomplish if the proper dietary cornerstones were in place? The solution might be found in the next chapter, where we examine the complex tango between nutrition and chronic illness, where each bite can either be a step toward recovery or a step toward worsening health problems.

You are still on your path to becoming an expert in managing Chronic Fatigue Syndrome, and together, we will skillfully and resolutely navigate its many facets.

Navigating Diets and Trends

The role of nutrition and diet is crucial in the intricate management of Chronic Fatigue Syndrome (CFS) and cannot be overstated. With diets and food trends blossoming like spring blossoms, the culinary landscape of today is as volatile as it is varied, with some offering the promise of life and others possessing the fragility of a passing fad.

I, Dr. Ankita Kashyap, offer my hand as your tour guide to help you navigate this maze of dietary options. Together, we will identify what really transforms individuals with CFS, not just what is trendy.

You may question, though, why we bring up diets while talking about CFS. The reasoning is based on the knowledge that our diets have the power to either aggravate or mitigate the symptoms of this mysterious illness. Our goal is to make it easier for you to make nutritional decisions that complement your body's particular requirements.

Let's set certain benchmarks for this investigation: nutritional balance, sustainability, and effectiveness in managing symptoms. These will be our waypoints as we navigate the waters of dietetics.

In today's health-conscious world, consider two dietary titans: the plant-based diet and the ketogenic diet. What do they have in common? Both have devoted fans who vouch for their transformative powers and promote cutting back on processed foods in favour of whole, nutrient-dense foods.

However, when we compare different diets, their differences stand out as much as day and night. The plant-based diet's celebration of fruits, vegetables, legumes, and grains contrasts sharply with the ketogenic diet's high-fat, moderate-protein, low-carb approach.

For a moment, consider how these diets would affect the body in the setting of CFS. One potential benefit of the ketogenic diet could be blood sugar stabilisation and a decreased inflammatory response. On the other hand, the plant-based diet is praised for having a high fibre content and a wealth of antioxidants, which are both beneficial in the battle against weariness caused by CFS.

However, what do these distinctions show? They emphasise that there is no one-size-fits-all treatment for CFS due to its complexity. The more general conclusion is evident: treating CFS calls for a customised strategy that takes into account a person's lifestyle, food preferences, and medical background.

Let us now move from theory to the real world that we live in. For patients with chronic fatigue syndrome (CFS), the popularity of "superfoods" and the appeal of "detox" diets are more than just passing trends; they symbolise optimism and the possibility of regaining their vigour. However, we must proceed with caution in this area because the allure of a fast fix may divert us from the road of long-term wellness.

I want you to be inquisitive and discerning as we look about this area. When a new diet or trend is offered, consider whether it meets our predetermined standards. Will it help my body fight chronic fatigue syndrome (CFS)?

Recall that achieving wellness is a marathon, not a sprint. And your best friends in this race will be persistence and patience.

Thus, as we get to the end of this chapter, my dear reader, I'd like you to consider this: Could it be that, in the vast scheme of CFS care, the secret to achieving your utmost well-being is not found in following dietary rules but rather in the delicate practise of listening—to your body, to science, and to the quiet wisdom that murmurs within?

We will continue this conversation in more detail in the next chapters as we examine nutrition's role in managing chronic fatigue syndrome (CFS) with the scientific method's accuracy and the healer's compassion. Together, we will plot a course that is guided by the unwavering stars of holistic wellbeing and individual empowerment rather than the whimsy of dietary trends.

Come along with me as we set out on this journey towards equilibrium and revitalization, where each mouthful has the capacity to cure and each meal is a step toward conquering Chronic Fatigue Syndrome.

Mental Health and Emotional Well-being

The Emotional Toll of CFS

The Emotional Toll of CFS

Have you ever experienced the thick, unrelenting invisible webs of tiredness that make getting out of bed seem like a monumental undertaking? Chronic fatigue syndrome, or CFS, is more than just a physical illness. It is a sneaky thief of life, a predatory condition that feeds on a person's emotional health. However, what if I told you that treating CFS's physical symptoms isn't the only aspect of managing it?

It is important to realise that CFS is not a standalone disorder as we explore its maze-like symptoms. It throws a shadow over all aspects of a person's life and frequently leaves a path of emotional upheaval in its wake. The fight is not just against exhaustion but also against the accompanying feelings of deep loss, dread, and frustration.

The conventional wisdom advises people with CFS to just take it easier and maybe go past their comfort zones, but this approach merely scratches the surface of a far more difficult problem. It ignores the intricate relationship that exists between mental and physical health, as well as between emotional and physical suffering.

But I encourage you to think about an alternative course that welcomes a comprehensive approach to CFS management. These pages include a blueprint, a paradigm change that recognises the complex relationships between your bodily and emotional states.

For a little period, see the burden of persistent fatigue not as a death sentence but rather as an opportunity for change. How do you discover clarity when tiredness turns everything around you into a blur? How can you get back the energy that CFS has taken from your life?

There isn't a single medication or treatment that works for everyone. It is woven through a complex web of dietary planning, lifestyle adjustments, and psychological support. In my capacity as a physician and health coach, I have seen innumerable patients undergo transformations as they learn to gracefully and powerfully traverse the turbulent waves of chronic tiredness.

Together, let's set out on a road that starts with admitting the emotional cost of CFS. It's time to stop doing what the majority of people do, which is to ignore the emotional fallout, and start paving the way for emotional empowerment and resilience.

The true answer is in going deeper, removing the emotional layers of distress to reveal the resilience that lies at the heart of each and every person living with CFS. By means of counselling, self-care routines, and coping mechanisms, we might amass an armamentarium to counter the affective consequences of this illness.

My method focuses on nurturing your full being rather than just treating your symptoms. Illness's about designing a life that works with CFS, but not letting it define you. With the correct techniques, you may learn to survive in spite of your sickness since you are not your condition.

This is a personal journey. It is evidence of your inner strength, which is frequently unrealized and eclipsed by the physical effects of CFS. As we proceed down this path, keep in mind that experiencing an emotional toll does not indicate weakness but rather a call to action and an opportunity to interact with your health on a more profound level.

Let me describe to you what life is like when you're not tired. Imagine a day when the chronic fatigue veil partways and you see the colours of passion and joy that CFS has dimmed. This vision is not a far-off dream; rather, it is a possible reality that starts with recognising and treating the emotional effects of your illness.

I so urge you to interact with your emotions as well as your intellect when you turn the pages of this book. Give yourself permission to experience the feelings that come up since they are your compass for healing. Accept the laughter, the tears, and the frustration as necessary components of the healing process.

And never forget, reader, that you possess a resilience stronger than your weariness. Your emotional mastery journey allows you to reclaim a part of yourself that CFS had hidden with each step.

As we get to the end of this chapter, take a moment to consider CFS's emotional journey. It's a difficult road, but one that will lead to significant personal development. Spread the word that you are capable of handling both the physical and emotional aspects of managing CFS, and that you have the means to do so.

We will delve deeper into these tools in the upcoming chapters and develop a holistic plan that addresses all facets of your health. Together, we will lay the groundwork for a life free from the limitations of chronic fatigue syndrome by constructing a foundation of resiliency, strength, and optimism.

Counseling and Therapy

Navigating the Mind's Maze in Chronic Fatigue Syndrome

Envision, if you will, a mental maze, with each turn signifying the intricate difficulties experienced by individuals suffering from Chronic Fatigue Syndrome (CFS). Imagine now that there is a beacon guiding these spirits through the maze, offering them support and clarity. The key to controlling the psychological elements of CFS is this beacon, which is the essence of counselling and therapy. I cordially invite you to go with me, Dr. Ankita Kashyap, as we delve into the core of this subchapter—the transformational potential of professional psychological support.

Let us shed light on the journey via the experiences of 34-year-old Maya, a graphic artist whose life was completely flipped upside down upon receiving a diagnosis of CFS. Maya felt lost in her own life as her vivid creativity was obscured by crippling exhaustion and disorganised thinking.

Maya's situation is not unusual. The primary obstacle she encountered was not alone the somatic manifestations of CFS, but also the psychological toll it took on her identity. She struggled with sadness, anxiety, and a strong sense of loneliness. The question was raised: how could she escape this syndrome's grip and take back her life?

Maya's healing path was initiated by a kind counsellor with expertise in chronic illness. They started a treatment journey together that included acceptance and commitment therapy, mindfulness exercises, and cognitive-behavioral therapy (CBT) (ACT). These techniques were designed specifically to assist Maya in navigating the psychological effects of CFS, changing the way she felt about the illness.

The outcomes were encouraging. Maya noted a notable decrease in her anxiety levels and an enhancement in her ability to cope with everyday exhaustion. She started to feel delight again in her art, something that had seemed like a faraway memory before. Her mood and coping skills demonstrated a positive rise, according to data from her therapy sessions, providing a qualitative and quantitative picture of her progress.

In retrospect, Maya's situation highlights the critical role that psychological support plays in helping people with CFS. It emphasises the significance of treating the mind-body connection and the usefulness of individualised therapy approaches. However, it is important to recognise that therapy is only one component of the intricate puzzle that is CFS care and is not a one-size-fits-all solution.

Maya's mood charts and fatigue diaries, among other visual aids, provided tangible evidence of her experience and insights for the CFS community at large as well as for herself. These resources illustrated the cyclical character of her symptoms and the progressive advantages of her treatment.

By relating Maya's storey to the broader storey of CFS care, it is evident how important it is to have expert counselling and therapy. They go beyond the simple symptom relief to promote a comprehensive sense of well-being, acting as the compass that points to empowerment and hope.

Have the entangling effects of chronic fatigue also caught you? Have you ever questioned if the mind plays an equally important role in your condition as the body does?

Give yourself permission to reflect for a moment. Think about the value of a helping hand as you navigate the psychological maze that is CFS. Imagine working together with a counsellor who is able to relate to you on a deeper level than just listening.

In summary, Maya's storey is a beacon of hope rather than merely a case study. It is a monument to the resiliency of the human spirit and serves as an example of the transformative power of counselling and therapy in the context of CFS.

As we get to the end of this section, I want to leave you with a question that I hope will ring in your mind: How may the light of psychological support have guided your own experience with CFS? Allow the response to this query to serve as the secret to opening a new chapter in your journey toward conquering chronic fatigue syndrome.

Keep in mind that the maze is a puzzle that needs to be solved rather than a prison as you proceed. And you possess the pieces here, dear reader, within these pages.

Building a Support System

Imagine being in the middle of an unrelenting storm with unwavering winds and a permanently dismal sky. Imagine a safe haven where a circle of helping hands is waiting to support you when things get chaotic. For people enduring the storm of chronic fatigue syndrome, that haven is the foundation of a strong support network (CFS).

Navigating a maze with no end in sight is how the experience with CFS is like. It's more than just being weary; it's a pervasive exhaustion that robs one of their own life force, exacerbated by a whirlwind of symptoms that can make it difficult to find the way back to health. The main obstacle? a constant sense of being alone, as if one were drifting in a sea of misinformation and doubt.

If left untreated, this isolation can have a domino effect that deteriorates symptoms, causes mental health issues, and causes a deep detachment from the world that was previously full of possibilities. Though not set in stone, it's a bleak scene. The power of connection to create a support system that functions as an anchor and compass is the remedy.

So how does one weave this essential support tapestry? Open communication is the first step. Talk to your loved ones not out of desperation but with the goal of enlightening them. Inform them about CFS, let them in on your reality, and let them know what you need, both practically and emotionally.

With bravery, move forward and strike up a discussion. Have you communicated to others around you the full scope of your experience? Have you allowed them to experience your life and learn what it's like to live with CFS?

Reach out to support groups, both online and in person, while you create this understanding bridge. You'll feel at home here with individuals who have experienced similar turbulent times and who are fluent in the CFS language. This common experience serves as a reminder that you are not travelling alone and is a source of strength.

Imagine now combining these links to create a coherent system. Start by naming important people in your life who can fulfil various functions. Some can be pillars of emotional support, while others might be skilled at helping with everyday chores. Maintain a schedule of frequent check-ins to ensure that these relationships are maintained. Recall that receiving help is a two-way street; your experiences can operate as a lighthouse and your insights as a road map for others.

However, what is the proof for the effectiveness of a support system? Research has demonstrated that social support can result in enhanced quality of life, decreased stress, and better health outcomes. One important factor in the management of CFS is a person's sense of control over their disease, which is something that people with strong networks frequently report having.

However, it is important to recognise that not everyone has access to a pre-existing support system. Alternative solutions beckon in these situations. With the help of telemedicine counselling, virtual support groups, and apps that link people with chronic illnesses, technology can close gaps in care. The secret is to continue being proactive and look for these resources with the same tenacity as managing any other element of CFS.

Building a support network takes time and care; it is not something that can be done quickly. It's like tending a garden: every relationship is a seed that can grow into a source of comfort and support if given the right care.

So, my reader, let's sow these seeds together. Together, with open communication, a common experience, and a strong dedication to connection, let's foster them. Because there is a profound truth hidden in this garden: working with CFS is not a lonely endeavour.

Numerous people have supported our journey, which is evidence of the human spirit's tenacity.

Take with you the commitment to create your support network as well as the knowledge of how to do so when you turn the page. Let this be the chapter that signals a change in direction, when the storm starts to pass and the sky becomes more likely to have sunny days ahead.

Dealing With Isolation and Loneliness

The gnawing feelings of loneliness and isolation are a struggle that those of us with Chronic Fatigue Syndrome (CFS) never talk about but feel deeply when we have quiet periods of repose as the world keeps on its unrelenting whirlwind outside our windows.

Imagine a world in which even the most basic pastimes, like going for a leisurely stroll or coffee with a buddy, become impossible chores. For many people with CFS, this is their everyday reality—a place where solitude may easily turn into a prison.

Loneliness presses not only on the spirit but also on the physical body. Isolation can lead to a host of health problems if left untreated, including decreased immune systems and deeper depression. Then, the question becomes: How can we recognise our bodies' need for rest while still reclaiming our feeling of community and connection?

The strength of creativity and intentionality in our interactions holds the key to the solution. Together, let's set out to create a path that will lead from the quiet into a place where even the most worn-out can experience the comfort of human connection.

The first step in realising this vision is to use technology as an ally. We now have a plethora of platforms thanks to the digital age that allow us to communicate with others from the comfort of our homes. For example, online support groups provide a forum for discussing common experiences as well as the understanding and affirmation that come from talking to others who have followed a similar route.

However, communication is not the only way that people connect. Even more potent can be the silent companionship of a video conference in which all parties are there but no one speaks, or the shared silence of an online meditation session.

All you really need to implement these digital interactions is a gadget and an internet connection. However, the results are significant. According to studies, people who participate in online communities report feeling far less alone, which is followed by a revitalised sense of purpose and belonging.

Virtual interactions are very useful, but nothing compares to the physical touch. Small, energy-efficient get-togethers can soothe lonely spirits for those who are capable of them. A quick visit from a friend or relative that is planned with boundaries to honour one's energy capacity can make the day happier and more upbeat.

Don't underestimate the influence of snail letter, though. A care box or a handwritten letter can fill the void left by distance and health limitations by serving as a concrete reminder that someone out there is thinking about you.

Naturally, there is no one-size-fits-all route to connection. The unconditional love and presence of a furry friend who provides comfort without requiring social graces or conversation can be a source of solace for some people.

Others might find that using their artistic mediums to express themselves—whether it be writing, painting, or music—makes them feel more connected to the outside world and builds a bridge to the hearts and minds of others.

The route out of solitude is ultimately quite personal. Patience, self-compassion, and the guts to reach out in the way that seems most genuine are necessary. We may start to re-weave the strands of connection into our lives by making these tiny, courageous moves, which will result in a tapestry full of hope, community, and support.

Therefore, to those of you who might experience the icy grip of isolation, know that the world is waiting for you outside of your four walls. Dare to connect, reach out, and tell those who can relate to your experience. And never forget that you are not alone, even in the silence of repose.

In conclusion, there is no easy way for those with CFS to overcome feelings of loneliness and isolation. However, we may return to a life filled with the relationships that keep us going by embracing technology, cultivating meaningful relationships, enjoying the joys of creativity and pets, and perhaps just taking a moment to relax and enjoy a peaceful visit. Let us find solace in the fact that we can manage to be together and apart during this difficult trip.

Mindfulness and Acceptance

The Art of Living Well with Chronic Fatigue Syndrome

Envision a world in which your body is an endless supply of energy and you wake up every morning feeling energised. Compare that to the reality that many people live with today—a world where Chronic Fatigue Syndrome (CFS) lurks like a silent thief taking one's life force. We will investigate the transforming potential of acceptance and mindfulness here, in this sacred space—the twin lights that help us see through the mist of exhaustion.

Imagine Jane, a once-burgeoning graphic artist, whose life unexpectedly took a turn for the worst when CFS engulfed her. An unbeatable battle was presented by the never-ending tiredness, the aches that seeped into her muscles, and the fog that obscured her once-alert thoughts.

As Jane's body begged for relief, the main battle she was facing became evident: how could she ever feel normal again? Jane found her refuge in the embrace of acceptance and mindfulness; the conventional medical route offered little consolation.

I introduced Jane to the concept of mindfulness, which is the discipline of living in the present moment with compassion and nonjudgment. We set out on a journey together to integrate mindfulness into her everyday life. Jane discovered how to accept her experiences, find a way to breathe through the pain, and pay attention to her feelings and thoughts without letting them control her.

We added the accepting principle to mindfulness. This was an admission of CFS's existence rather than a white flag of capitulation. Jane discovered her boundaries and learnt to pay attention to her body's warning signals before they turned into screaming. Rather than reacting with resistance and irritation, she took a calm, inquisitive approach to her symptoms.

Although the changes took time to manifest, the effects were obvious. Jane started to develop a healthy connection with her body. She changed her activities in response to her energy's ups and downs. Even on her worst days, she found moments of happiness and fulfilment.

Patients like Jane who practised acceptance and mindfulness reported a significant decrease in the perceived burden of their symptoms, according to data from our clinic. They spoke of an improved standard of living, a stronger sense of self, and the capacity to face challenges head-on and bounce back.

Thinking back on situations such as Jane's, it is clear that although CFS can be an obstinate opponent, mental strength can be a powerful friend. Although they are not miracle cures, acceptance and mindfulness are powerful tools in the toolbox of anyone trying to live well with CFS.

Patients are provided with a concrete means of incorporating mindfulness into their everyday routines through visual aids like breathing exercises and audio recordings of guided meditations.

The storey of this book echoes the wider ramifications of Jane's path toward acceptance and awareness. These approaches are more than just coping mechanisms; they offer a route to self-actualization and empowerment for individuals managing the intricacies of long-term sickness.

As we come to the end of this chapter, I'd want to leave you with this concept to consider, dear reader: How may the subtle practise of acceptance and mindfulness light your path in your personal CFS journey, leading you toward a life defined by mastery over exhaustion rather than by constant struggle?

Recognizing your inner strength to be present, accept, and turn suffering into strength is the first step toward managing Chronic Fatigue Syndrome completely. I hope this mastery bible provides you with comfort, tips, and most importantly, hope as you flip the pages.

Boosting Self-Esteem and Confidence

In the complex process of coping with Chronic Fatigue Syndrome (CFS), we frequently fail to see a subtle but potent foe: the decline in confidence and self-worth. In my capacity as a physician and wellness coach, I have personally observed the unwavering perseverance of those battling this illness. However, I've also witnessed the self-assurance light go out in their eyes. It is a crisis of silence, rumbling doubts and anxieties that, if ignored, can burst into a gulf of hopelessness.

What is the main obstacle in this situation? It's the sneaky notion that having CFS limits makes one less valuable. This condition has the potential to alter one's sense of self, resulting in an inaccurate assessment of one's value and ability. Such a mindset has far-reaching ramifications that might threaten one's identity at its core, ranging from social seclusion to a reluctance to pursue personal ambitions.

However, hope is present. Evidence-based, pragmatic tactics that can boost confidence and fan the flames of self-esteem are a beacon of light. To regain the ground lost to CFS, let's set out on a transforming journey.

Cognitive restructuring, a psychological strategy that involves recognising and challenging negative thought patterns and substituting them with more balanced and constructive ones, is the cornerstone of the treatment. By taking this stance, people can reframe their experiences with CFS so that they are seen as challenges that can be overcome with grace and resiliency rather than as unsurmountable barriers.

Keep a diary as you start to weave this tapestry of change. Write down any negative beliefs you may have about yourself every day, and then refute them with proof of your accomplishments and intrinsic worth, no matter how minor they may seem. Have you brought a smile on someone's face today? Note it down. Have you succeeded in reading a few pages of a book? Let's celebrate it. These little victories added together might create a stronghold of one's own value.

The exercise of self-compassion is another essential component. Be kind and understanding to yourself as you would a close friend. Remind yourself that it's acceptable to take breaks, withdraw, and take care of your body and soul when exhaustion sweeps over you like a relentless tide.

Take part in things that make you happy and give you a sense of achievement. Painting, gardening, and crafts are examples of non-trivial pursuits that connect you to your soul and the core of who you are outside of CFS.

Ever thought about how important posture is? Studies highlight the relationship that exists between our mental and bodily states. Breathe deeply while maintaining a tall posture and back shoulders. This small action might inform your brain that you are strong and prepared to take on the world.

The orchestra of social support is something we should not overlook. Those who support you, who can see past your condition, and who will celebrate each step you take should be in your immediate vicinity. This network will help you rebuild your self-esteem; it is not a crutch.

And keep in mind the stars at night. Even if they have nothing to do with your current situation, consider your earlier accomplishments. The battlefield may have changed, but the warrior inside of you still exists. You are still the one who accomplished those achievements.

Maybe you're asking yourself, "What if these strategies don't resonate with me?" That is a legitimate worry. Alternative approaches like seeking professional counselling or joining support groups can be quite helpful in these situations. Sometimes, just talking about your difficulties might make them seem less significant.

I've seen my patients' self-belief return through these many approaches. Once-dejected eyes now shine with determination. It is evidence of the ability of the human spirit to overcome hardship.

Finally, keep in mind that although CFS may have played a role in your life, it does not determine your value. Your sickness does not define who you are. Your potential is infinite and your worth is unchangeable. You recover a little bit of yourself with every stride ahead. So, my reader, take a stance and move forward. Mastering Chronic Fatigue Syndrome requires more than just treating symptoms; it also entails fostering self-belief and the conviction that you are and always will be enough.

Navigating Relationships With CFS

Navigating Relationships with CFS

Imagine finding yourself on a boat in the middle of a wide ocean when you wake up one day. Your body, this boat, is now vulnerable to the erratic waves of Chronic Fatigue Syndrome (CFS), a disorder as confusing as the ocean. Energy currents come and go suddenly, and those who used to be your friends, family, and crew could find it difficult to accompany you on these unfamiliar journeys. There is an unseen battle going on here that has the power to break even the strongest of relationships.

Chronic fatigue syndrome is a relationship test as much as a physical challenge. The greatest difficulty is sustaining closeness and connection when your physical and mental energy are always depleted. Family members could be put in strange parts, with relationships and expectations shifting under their feet like sand.

If the effects of CFS are not treated, they can cause miscommunication, animosity, and even a severe feeling of loneliness in your relationships. Not only can relationships suffer when a person has CFS; these connections also require care and support to be healthy.

So what is the solution in this kind of circumstance? The foundation of the bridge we need to construct is communication. Being open and truthful about your skills together with learning about CFS will help you develop patience and empathy in your inner circle. However, in an environment where energy is a valuable resource, how can we effectively communicate?

This is where "energy economy" art is found. Set work and social engagements as your top priorities to save energy for deep conversations. The quality that feeds the roots of a relationship, not the amount of time spent with loved ones, is what matters.

Now let's get into the specifics of putting successful communication methods into practise. Start by establishing firm yet sensitive limits. Something as simple as "I need to relax now; may we continue this later?" can be assertive and elegant. To help them comprehend the "why" behind your behaviours, educate your family and friends about CFS, maybe through resources you offer. Plan frequent check-ins to find out how everyone is handling the changes brought on by CFS. This might be done by setting up a family meeting or a weekly video call.

There is much proof of the effectiveness of effective communication. Families coping with long-term medical conditions report greater psychological health and stronger connections among all members after attending support groups and therapy sessions. It proves the proverb "a problem shared is a problem half."

What about other approaches? "Mindful presence" is a practise that can be very beneficial. When exhaustion prevents you from engaging in activities, savouring the little moments can foster enduring emotional bonds. A tender look, a squeeze of the hand, or a few exchanged words might mean a great deal.

In addition, technology can fill in the gaps in situations where being physically present is not possible. A shared photo, a text message, or an online game can sustain the spirit of friendship.

In my capacity as your tour guide, I beg you to think about: Do you take the same care with your relationships as you do with your own health?

As they say, "less is more," and this also applies to words. Select them carefully, judiciously, and lovingly. The most valuable resource in the communication economy is comprehension.

Relationships have a rhythm that's similar to music: a dynamic interaction of giving and receiving, speaking and remaining silent, and being there and not present. Make an effort to discover harmony in these beats, and allow your interactions to have a dancing tempo rather than a marching one.

I'd like to leave you with this thought: How may your experience with CFS change your relationships as well as yourself into something more meaningful, strong, and stunningly unexpected?

Relationships are the threads that bind us together in the fabric of life. Let us weave, even with tired hands, with attention to detail, patience, and slow, purposeful strokes. Ultimately, it is our collective power that enables us to confront the immense array of obstacles.

Lifestyle Modifications for CFS

Energy Conservation Techniques

For a brief instant, picture the energy that used to flow through your veins. With Chronic Fatigue Syndrome (CFS), it appears to be a thing of the past. The pursuit of energy turns into a journey as unrelenting as the seas. But what if I told you that you could navigate these waters with a newfound elegance if you had the appropriate map? We will set off on just such a journey in this important subchapter, laying out a plan for efficient energy conservation—a ray of hope amidst the exhaustion.

Establish the Goal

If you accept the challenge, your goal is to become an expert in energy saving and reverse the chronic weariness that comes with CFS. One breath at a time, you are recovering the essence of your strength; you are not just getting by every day.

List the Necessary Materials or Prerequisites

Make sure you have a few necessities in your toolkit before we go: an open heart prepared for transformation, a journal for monitoring and reflection, and a readiness to adopt new habits. Above all, you will use patience as a compass to navigate the waves of change.

Begin with a Broad Overview

The general stages of energy management—identifying energy drains, setting priorities, mastering pace, and putting restorative activities into practice—mark the start of our journey. Every element on our map serves as a crucial waypoint.

Dive into Detailed Steps

Recognizing Energy Drains

First, list in your journal the things that drain your energy. This could involve strenuous physical activity, stressful situations, or even food decisions. Are you noticing any trends? This knowledge serves as a lighthouse to steer clear of energy-draining shoals.

Prioritizing Tasks

Let's go ahead and prioritise your tasks. What needs to get done today and what can wait? It's an easy but meaningful gesture that enables you to plan your day and save your energy for the things that really count.

Learning Pacing Techniques

Your constant current is your pacing. Discovering the cadence that permits you to manoeuvre through your day without colliding with the boulder of fatigue is the key. Divide the work into smaller, more manageable waves and space out the waves with brief breaks. You'll stay afloat with this ebb and flow.

Implementing Restorative Practices

Lastly, we use activities that refuel us to anchor our day. This may be deep breathing, meditation, or light exercise—anything that stills the raging oceans inside you and enables your body to heal and regenerate itself.

Offer Tips and Warnings

Take care not to sail too close to the wind when you set out on this adventure. Overdoing it can result in a relapse, and disobeying your body's cues might leave you lost. Learn to say no, and always keep in mind that sleep is your life preserver, not a luxury.

Testing or Validation

When you successfully preserve energy, how will you know? It's all documented in your journal. Take note of your weariness changes and the environment surrounding them. Gradually, an enhanced energy pattern will show you where you've come.

Troubleshooting (optional)

If you notice that you're drifting off course, go back and review your journal. If you find that certain activities wear you out, adjust your sails accordingly. This is a cue to adjust your strategy rather than a setback.

Have you ever stopped to thought about the potential of a single, concentrated breath? Take a deep breath in. You are replenishing your energy now, right now. Energy conservation is a philosophy and a way of life, not just a set of behaviours.

I beg you to take a moment to consider the journey thus far as we come to the end of this chapter. Energy conservation is a sail that catches the winds of change, not an anchor that drags you down. You are not just coping with CFS; you are becoming adept at it with every step, guiding your life toward a future full of energy and promise.

Recall that the journey towards energy conservation is a marathon rather than a sprint. May you find the fortitude to run it with grace and endurance by using the strategies and insights offered in these pages. Hold this book near at hand, much like a reliable compass, and consult it frequently while you continue to navigate the wide sea of life with CFS.

As the sun sets on this trip, dear reader, know that every new dawn offers the chance to sail a little more smoothly, save a little more energy, and live a little fuller. This is a chapter in your life storey, not just a chapter in a book. Write it with excellence.

Sleep Hygiene Practices

Your Pathway to Restorative Slumber

Have you ever sat in bed and stared at the ceiling, wishing against hope that sleep would come over you, only to have it elude you? You're not alone if you're nodding wistfully in accord. Finding healing sleep might seem like a Sisyphean chore for people suffering from Chronic Fatigue Syndrome (CFS). But have no fear—I, Dr. Ankita Kashyap, am here to lead you through the sacred corridors of sleep hygiene and turn your bedroom into a peaceful haven.

Our goal is straightforward but profound: by promoting good sleep hygiene, we hope to help people suffering with CFS enter a new phase of rest and recuperation.

To embark on this nocturnal odyssey, you'll need a few essentials:
- A sleep diary for tracking your progress.
- Comfortable bedding that beckons you to rest.
- A quiet, dark, and cool environment.
- A heart willing to embrace new routines.

Now let's unfold the action plan that will take us to the promised land of sound slumber. Setting a sleep schedule is the first step in our trip. From there, we'll explore how to create the perfect sleeping environment, participate in pre-slumber rituals, and end with daily habits that respect the night.

1. Set a Sleep Schedule: The secret is to be consistent, just like a maestro leading an orchestra. Yes, even on the weekends, retire and get up at the same hours every day. Regularity is vital to your body's internal clock, a sensitive watch.

2. Create Your Sleep Sanctuary: Your bedroom ought to evoke feelings of peace and quiet. Devices that emit the blue glow of consciousness should be banished. Cover your windows with black cloth. Keep the night breeze lulling you into slumber and the air cool.

3. Pre-Slumber Rituals: Your pace should slow as dusk approaches. Reduce the brightness to let your mind know that the moment of consciousness is almost here. Take up some soft hobbies, like reading a nice book, taking a warm bath, or writing a sonnet to yourself.

4. Honor the Day, Embrace the Night: Allow the light of day to follow you about, as exercise leads to the delightful yielding of exhaustion. However, you should cut back on your coffee and substantial meals as the sun sets. Give the night control over both activity and nourishment.

- A word to the wise: Alcohol and sleep aids are like sirens that lure you in with their promises of ease but only give you broken sleep. If at all, use them sparingly.

- Consider the lullaby of white noise or earplugs if silence eludes you.

How will you know whether the fabric of good sleep hygiene that you've knitted together holds? Your sleep journal will document the patterns that appear and the change in sleep quality from restless to peaceful nights. Refreshed—a feeling that might have faded into the past—you'll awaken.

Don't worry if Morpheus still seems like an erratic friend. Changes are possible. Maybe you should adjust your timetable or sanctify your surroundings more. Your allies are perseverance and patience.

Now, my reader, let us set forth into the sacred night with the map ingrained in our minds and the compass of commitment at our disposal. I pray that the stars overhead will witness your journey to a peaceful place to sleep and that the energy of the night will fill your days with colour.

You can achieve sleep, that elusive conundrum that many with Chronic Fatigue Syndrome struggle to achieve. This is a journey of perseverance rather than an overnight odyssey. If you stick with these routines, eventually the sleep puzzle pieces will fit together to create a mosaic of vigour and renewal.

Never forget, my dear traveller, that the night is a friend to be welcomed rather than an enemy to be vanquished. Your bed is a place of healing, not a battlefield. This subchapter is just the start of your adventure. You'll discover a wealth of techniques in "The Chronic Fatigue Syndrome Mastery Bible: Your Blueprint for Complete Chronic Fatigue Syndrome Management" that go beyond sleep and are all intended to support you on your journey to wellness.

Let the last thought you have before falling asleep tonight be one of hope, because this book contains the steps to not only manage but also truly master chronic fatigue syndrome. Good night, and may you have pleasant dreams that are finally within your grasp.

Creating a Restorative Environment

Have you ever thought about how much your environment affects your health? Picture a peaceful haven where you may feel renewed energy coursing through your tired bones. This is a world that is within your reach, not some far-off ideal. A crucial first step toward treating Chronic Fatigue Syndrome is to turn your house into a healing refuge. Let's go on this adventure together (CFS).

Our goal is straightforward yet profound: to create a space that supports your healing and tranquilly. In addition to relieving your symptoms, this healing environment will strengthen your resistance to the ups and downs of CFS.

Make sure you have an open mind, a desire to embrace change, and a dash of imagination before we move forward. assemble physical comforts like cosy blankets, tranquil aromatherapy aromas, and calming hues. Prepare your area for clearing out clutter and bring peace into every corner.

The road map to creating a healing space includes organising your belongings, selecting the ideal colour scheme, maximising lighting, adding greenery, customising your sleeping haven, and adding sentimental touches.

Let's take a closer look at decluttering. Start by taking a compassionate yet firm look through your possessions and retaining only the things that fulfil you or make you happy. Creating a stress-free environment starts with a clutter-free space.

Let's discuss about colour next. The colours you choose for your walls and furniture should exude tranquilly. Select hues that convey a sense of life and tranquilly, such as muted earth tones, warm greens, or light blues.

Now think about the lighting. Let the natural light fill your room; it's a soul-saving cure. Select artificial lighting sources that emulate natural light sources rather than harsh fluorescent ones.

Dimmer switches let you customise the atmosphere to your preferred level of comfort.

Integrate natural elements to bring the outside in. Your little indoor fountain or a few potted plants might work wonders for your mental haven. There is something intrinsically healing about being in nature.

Your bedroom, your haven of rest, needs extra care. Purchase supportive pillows and a high-quality mattress to enhance your sleep. When you need to recharge, blackout curtains can screen you from the outside world, and a white noise machine can block out distracting noises.

Finally, add your unique touch. A bookcase filled with your favourite books or pictures that bring back pleasant memories can add personality and a sense of inner space to your room.

When you start this project, be careful not to overstimulate. Overindulgence in ornamentation or clashing patterns can strain the eyes. Strive for harmony and simplicity.

Recall that scents ought to be reassuring rather than overbearing. To be sure essential oils don't cause symptoms, test little amounts of them.

Once these adjustments are put into place, evaluate your space's emotional resonance. Does it encourage you to unwind? As you walk in, do you notice that your breath gets deeper? These indicate that your surroundings and your healing process are in sync.

If you are still feeling overburdened or worn out, go over each component again. It might need to be adjusted. Maybe the lighting needs to be adjusted, or the colours need to be softer. Let your space change with you because it is a mirror of your inner condition.

Your house can either support or deplete you in the dance of light and shade. Carrying the awareness torch, you've discovered how to create a space that supports your road to wellness by existing around you and interacting with you.

Recall, my dear reader, that although the path to managing chronic fatigue syndrome is complex and frequently difficult, every action you take to establish a restorative environment is a step toward recovering your energy. The book "The Chronic Fatigue Syndrome Mastery Bible: Your Blueprint for Complete Chronic Fatigue Syndrome Management" contains much more information than this subchapter does. It's evidence of the holistic philosophy I like, which weaves together the elements of environment, mind, body, and spirit to create a healing and hopeful tapestry.

I hope that as you flip each page, you will discover wisdom, courage, and most importantly, a friend in your quest for wellbeing. Cheers to mastering your journey one breath at a time, one space at a time, and one moment at a time.

Exercise and Activity Management

The Pacing Paradox

Imagine waking up each morning with your thoughts clouded, muscles hurting, and exhaustion from recently finishing a marathon. For people suffering from chronic fatigue syndrome, this is their everyday life (CFS). But let me ask you, what if the same thing that appears to be at odds with your illness turns out to be a key component of your therapeutic approach? Yes, I do mean activity and exercise, but not in the traditional sense. It's time to investigate the fine tango between effort and recuperation, to discover a balance that promotes your health without tipping the scales in favour of relapse.

The paradox is that, although rest is crucial, inactivity can worsen physical health and, in a cruel twist of irony, exacerbate CFS symptoms. The difficulty lies not in idleness per se, but in how it is managed, and the fallout from poor management is far from insignificant. Imagine the boom-bust cycle, which consists of days of crippling exhaustion after excessive exertion. This pattern is all too common and depressing for many who suffer from CFS.

Our answer is right here: pace. This approach is about learning to pay attention to your body's signals and adapting your exercise and activity routine accordingly, not about placing restrictions on yourself. Pacing involves taking deliberate, modest actions that respect your existing capabilities and gradually push your bounds over time.

Understanding your baseline—what you can do on a poor day without making your symptoms worse—is the first step in putting pacing into practise. From here, we gradually up the amount of activity while continuously paying attention to the body's signals. It's a process of trial and error, and failures are only useful lessons to help you improve your strategy.

Pacing has been shown to be effective beyond anecdotal evidence. Research has indicated that CFS symptoms can be alleviated with carefully controlled activity, proving that the appropriate type and quantity of exercise can improve quality of life without causing the dreaded post-exercisional malaise.

But what if you find that pacing isn't effective? It is conceivable. Our responses to CFS are as different from one another as our fingerprints are. Other options include cognitive behavioural treatment (CBT) and graded exercise therapy (GET), both of which have demonstrated efficacy in some patients. These techniques are not without debate, though, so they should be used carefully and under expert advice.

How therefore do we start incorporating exercise into our daily lives without creating a fabric of exhaustion? Take it slow at first, a little stroll or some light stretching, and pay attention. How does your body respond? What is your mood the following day? The secret is to be consistent without going overboard.

Isn't it ironic that for those with CFS, moving about may be both a remedy and a poison? Absolutely. However, there is hope for improved symptom management within this contradiction.

Every conscious action moves one closer to empowerment. And isn't that the main objective? to take back control of our life storey from CFS?

I'd want to leave you with this concept to consider as we wrap up this chapter: Is it possible for the knowledge of pace to change your experience with CFS from one of grace to one of endurance? The next chapter of your life is entirely up to you, but know that you are not travelling this route alone. Step by step, one timed step at a time, we walk together towards a life that is not defined by weariness but rather by the abundance of experiences we can still embrace.

Time Management and Prioritization

Harnessing Your Energy Wisely

A fundamental truth that is frequently discovered during the tortuous process of managing Chronic Fatigue Syndrome (CFS) is that time management is not only a talent but a profound art. The ability to prioritise tasks and manage your time effectively becomes essential as you move through your days while carrying the weight of your fluctuating energy levels. This subsection serves as your road map to that creativity, a step-by-step guide to balancing your schedule with your energy.

Here, we are all on a singular mission: to provide you with the tools necessary to synchronise your everyday responsibilities with the erratic energy waves that CFS brings. The goal, my dear reader, is to turn time into a canvas, filling your days with endeavours that honour your energy reserves while also adding a feeling of fulfilment to your existence.

You will require a diary or digital planner, a thorough comprehension of your present energy patterns, and an openness to embrace flexibility in order to begin this journey. Embrace an open mind and a dedication to self-compassion as you discover how to dance with your day instead of rushing through it.

First, let's take a look at what lies ahead: we will determine your energy patterns, set priorities, and design a flexible plan. These three actions will be the cornerstones of your temple dedicated to time management.

1. Start by monitoring your energy levels for a fortnight. Make a note of the times of day that you are the most energetic and the ones that are dominated by exhaustion. It is this self-awareness that will serve as your daily compass.

2. Make a list of your tasks, separating "must-do" from "nice-to-do," using your energy patterns as a guide. Which tasks are

essential to your health and which ones might you potentially postpone or delegate? This discernment is the cornerstone around which your everyday routine will be constructed.

3. In this section, your priorities and your energy insights are combined. Plan more strenuous activities for when your energy is at its highest and lighter, less strenuous activities for when it is at its lowest. Make time for unplanned rest periods and sudden low energy.

- Have a realistic outlook. The enemy of CFS management is overcommitment.

Pay attention to your body. If there isn't a scheduled task for today, it's an act of self-care rather than a defeat.

- Your ally is flexibility. Fixed schedules crack under the erratic weight of CFS; they are brittle.

You'll know you've created an effective plan when you go through the week with a sense of increased control, less hurry, and stamina for the important things. Instead of being a slave to the clock, you will become its composer, setting the time to suit your body's demands.

Reevaluate your energy patterns if you notice that your schedule and energy levels are consistently at odds; they might have changed. Keep in mind that CFS is a dynamic condition, thus your tactics need to be flexible too.

Now, let us delve deeper.

If you will, picture a day that is shaped by your own energy, gently and intelligently, rather than by the incessant ticking of the clock. Imagine how freeing that would be.

When you start tracking your energy (step 1), it's normal if at first you don't see any trends. CFS can be erratic, with varying symptoms. Even so, small patterns will start to show themselves. Write these down. Is there a strand of life visible in the morning silence? Or maybe an energy burst in the late afternoon that wasn't anticipated? These are the hours of gold to seize.

When you move on to step two, which is prioritising your chores, consider the following: What is actually necessary? Does the task keep your world turning, your soul nourished, or your health intact? Can it wait if not?

When you schedule (step three), picture your day as a symphony of notes. Your adagios are the low-energy chores, and your crescendos are the high-energy ones. What about the others? These are the score's rests—the pauses that offer the music nuance and balance to your day.

A piece of advise for the astute: resist the urge to pack your day with activities. Being spacious does not equate to being idle; rather, it is wise energy conservation.

My dear reader, are you feeling the change? the idea that time could not always be an enemy but rather an ally?

When confirming the effectiveness of your novel strategy through testing or validation, pay attention to how you feel at the end of the day. Has your activity had a rhythm that feels in line with your inner tempo, an ebb and flow? That is a definite indication of mastery.

And if difficulties (troubleshooting) come up, keep trying. Have the willingness to revise, rewrite, and discard your plans. Like you, your planner or notebook is a living document that is not static.

Finally, keep this in mind: For the CFS warrior, managing their time is about getting things done in the time they have, not about getting things done more. It's about realising the worth of every moment and your ability to influence it. When this chapter comes to an end and you look ahead to tomorrow's blank canvas, ask yourself, "What will my masterpiece look like?"

You are creating a life with every choice you make and every order in which you set priorities, not just managing time.

Adapting Work and Career

Imagine that the threads of ambition and purpose that weave your everyday existence together suddenly begin to fray, one by one. Who's at fault? Chronic fatigue syndrome (CFS) is an illness that gradually depletes your energy and leaves you feeling exhausted all the time, even when you're at rest.

Take some time to think as you flip through the pages of this booklet. Have you observed how CFS has affected your aspirations for your career and place of employment? The dreams you've worked so hard to create could gradually escape your grasp like grains of sand if left unchecked.

The main difficulty with the maze of CFS is that it is erratic and variable. Your energy is not only finite, but also unpredictable. You may feel strong when you wake up, but by midday, fatigue may catch you off guard. It is possible for conventional work structures to feel like a square peg in a round hole because of this erratic energy distribution.

What would happen if we ignored this challenge? The ramifications extend well beyond our careers. Failing to modify our careers to suit our new reality can lead to social isolation, financial difficulty, and a declining sense of self-worth.

However, let's avoid hanging out on the edge of hopelessness. Instead, let us examine a solution that not only shines brilliantly but can be achieved with the appropriate effort. This is a light of hope. The secret is to modify your job and profession to better suit your present skills. This entails rethinking your career with adaptability and self-compassion as its central ideas.

To begin putting this option into practise, have an open discussion with your employer. Being open and honest about your illness creates the foundation for cooperation and understanding. Next, plan out changes to your workload or schedule. Could you work from home or change to a part-time schedule? A flexible work schedule or job sharing can be the solution.

Research indicates that flexible work environments witness a rise in worker happiness and productivity. This is advantageous for business as well as for you.

Naturally, not every approach works for every situation. It may be necessary for certain people to shift careers. This is changing your passions to fit your new form, not giving up on them. It could entail learning new skills that enable you to work from the comforts of your own home or looking for jobs that are just as gratifying but less physically demanding.

Have you given self-employment any thought? This route has made it possible for many CFS sufferers to work in a more regulated setting. You establish the hours, the pace, and most importantly, the standards.

But first, let's take a brief break. Are there any additional options that we haven't considered? Support groups, where people share their experiences and develop innovative employment ideas catered to individuals with CFS, provide comfort to some. Some might discover that taking a break from work gives them the opportunity to recuperate and plan their next career move without the everyday demands of employment.

Remember that adaptation is a badge of bravery and inventiveness rather than a sign of weakness as you find yourself at the intersection of your work and health. Even while the future you choose might not be what you had in mind, it can still be quite fulfilling.

As we get to the end of this chapter, dear reader, consider the following: what actions can you do right now to make your professional life more in line with your health? Even with CFS, how can you start writing new goals that will make you happy, fulfilled, and feel like you've accomplished something?

The Chronic Fatigue Syndrome Mastery Bible is a travel companion that will help you regain control over your life, not just a guide. Let's work together to transform the difficulty of adjusting to a new job and career into an opportunity to redefine success and find your talents. After all, learning how to dance in the rain is a greater sign of expertise than never falling.

Traveling With CFS

Traveling with CFS

Have you ever experienced a conflicting desire for the calming touch of far-off beaches while also detesting the idea of making the necessary travels to get there? This chapter will help you heal from the wanderlust that has taken hold of you if you are nodding in tired agreement.

Establish the Goal:

Our goal is very clear: we want to travel with Chronic Fatigue Syndrome (CFS) and come out on the other side not only uninjured but also improved by the experience.

List the Necessary Materials or Prerequisites:

You will need a well-thought-out plan, a customised toolset of coping mechanisms, and a heart full of patience and self-compassion to embark on this path.

Begin with a Broad Overview:

Consider the procedure as a tapestry made of self-awareness, adaptability, and readiness. We'll plot our course, prepare our metaphorical "packs" with useful tips, and modify our sails according to the conditions.

Dive into Detailed Steps:

1. The journey starts in the solitude of your own thoughts long before you step outside. Plan an itinerary that offers ample time for each destination. Make time for relaxation days and choose lodgings that offer peace and quiet.

2. Your suitcase should be a veritable treasure trove of necessities, carrying only lightweight, manageable items that will keep you comfortable and nourished. Consider energy-boosting foods, noise-cancelling headphones, and comfortable travel pillows.

3. For people with CFS, airports can be energy vampires. To reduce layovers, choose for direct flights, request assistance in

advance, and think about lounge access for a more peaceful waiting area.

4. Allow the trip to play just as big of an influence as the final destination. You can take in the surroundings more slowly and save energy and tension by not rushing.

5. Pick pursuits that align with your level of energy. There's a chance that a peaceful beach sunset will nourish you more than any tourist excursion of the day.

6. Always keep a backup plan. Keep your prescriptions, medical records, and anything else that can help with unexpected symptom flare-ups in a tiny emergency kit.

Offer Tips and Warnings:

It is impossible to overstate how important it is to stay hydrated. The oil is what maintains the engine's smooth operation.

Adhere to the diet that you find most effective. It is not a good idea to try new meals while travelling since they might cause problems.

- The power of communication should never be undervalued. To make sure your travelling partners can assist you, let them know what you need.

- Keep medical records close to hand at all times. When your health takes an unexpected turn, you should be ready, not scared.

Validation or Testing:

When you can look back on your voyage with a heart full with memories and a sense of accomplishment rather than a body heavy with fatigue, you will know that you have successfully navigated your travels.

Troubleshooting:

Don't be afraid to change your plans if you notice a decline in your energy or a flare-up of your symptoms. It is quite OK to take a day off, switch to a less taxing activity, or, in extreme cases, consult a local physician.

—-

Let's now, dear reader, explore this travel-themed tapestry in more detail, with each thread holding the possibility of new learning and comprehension.

is more than just plans and timetables; it's about learning to feel your body's rhythm. When does it start singing with energy? When does it murmur to sleep? This innate understanding moulds your path.

is a mindfulness activity that goes beyond just what's in your suitcase. Every piece is a travel companion that you have selected for comfort and usefulness rather than glitz and beauty.

The beautiful dance of is similar to the art of. Every stage is planned, from boarding to security inspections, so you save your energy for the marvels that lie ahead.

is to pick the picturesque route instead of the busy one. It is putting oneself completely in the present and allowing each experience to permeate into who you are without feeling hurried.

You accept your limitations and acknowledge your advantages when making a decision. It's realising that happiness is in the richness of every moment rather than how many things you can cross off a list.

You are a comforter and a shield. It's the comforting murmur in your ear that says, "You are ready for any rising waters."

Recall that dealing with CFS requires patience; it's not a race. Not only is there a destination in the end, but also evidence of your perseverance. You go not as a warrior but as a sage, wise in the understanding of your own strength and the courage of your spirit, through the heights of delight and the lowlands of exhaustion.

Let the thought pass you by while you stand there, maybe in front of an ocean or on the edge of a cobblestone street in a distant land: you have travelled farther than just a few kilometres; you have travelled far within yourself.

In that quiet triumphant moment, remember that this chapter is only a portion of a broader discussion we are having about living with CFS, not just existing. So, no matter how far you have to travel, take these words, hold them close to your heart, and move forth with the assurance of someone who knows the way home.

Self-Help Techniques and Coping Strategies

Journaling and Self-Reflection

The Unseen Allies in Chronic Fatigue Syndrome Management

Imagine a haven hidden deep within your own head, a place where the echoes of your everyday difficulties and the whispering of your darkest thoughts are not only acknowledged but also understood. This is the domain of journaling and introspection, an area of therapeutic support for individuals suffering from Chronic Fatigue Syndrome (CFS). As Dr. Ankita Kashyap, I am excited to walk you through the healing potential of these tools since I have personally experienced their transformative impact.

Let's explore the life of Emily, a lively graphic designer whose diagnosis with CFS caused an unanticipated turn of events. The never-ending exhaustion, the mental fog, and the plethora of symptoms that followed her like shadows threatened to put a halt to her creative spirit.

Like many CFS patients, Emily found that the main challenges were not just the physical symptoms but also their psychological anguish and loneliness. The question arose: Is it possible to uncover a more tolerable existence with CFS through journaling and self-reflection?

Emily set out on her quest with kind encouragement, using her pen as a sceptre to defeat her unseen foe. The strategy involved two parts: a daily journal to record her experiences and focused introspection to identify the trends and triggers that led to her exhaustion.

The findings were instructive. Similar to constellations in the night sky, patterns started to emerge: stress, particular foods, and disturbed sleep were her enemies. However, there were also rays of hope; her entries started to highlight joyful and restorative pursuits.

Based on our investigation, these findings were crucial. They made it possible for us to customise Emily's care, improving her nutrition, quality of sleep, and coping mechanisms. Writing turned become a way for her to let go and a daily routine that gave her a sense of control over her situation.

Though they are not necessary in this situation, visual aids frequently enhance this kind of reflection. Graphs that show variations in mood or energy levels over time can be quite effective in pointing out personal patterns and stressors.

By tying these particulars back to the main storey, we can understand that journaling and introspection are journeys of self-discovery rather than just depressing diaries. They are the unsaid discourse that develops self-awareness and moves a person toward holistic healing between the body and the mind.

Now consider this: What revelations could be hidden within of you and only need to be uncovered by writing anything down?

Let's embrace language simplicity going forward to make sure our message is understood: Not only are journaling and self-reflection therapeutic activities, but they are also acts of self-care that have the capacity to shed light on the murky seas of CFS.

Think about Emily's experience. A pattern of coping became apparent through the cadence of her daily entries. Was it simple? Not every time. Was it worthwhile, though? Absolutely.

Using quotes, allow me to share with you an observation made by Anaïs Nin that Emily found to be quite true: "We write to taste life twice, in the moment and in retrospect." Emily recovered her life with CFS through journaling, not just documented it.

Let's acknowledge, finally, the clarity that arises from the introspective dance of journaling and the strength in vulnerability that results from self-reflection. These are our invisible partners in the fight against chronic fatigue syndrome.

I'll leave you with this transitional idea to consider as you turn the page: If you were to go on this path of self-discovery, how would your personal narrative change?

Cognitive Behavioral Techniques

Imagine experiencing a constant state of fatigue upon getting up each morning, making every movement seem like a monumental undertaking. This is the unrelenting situation that people with Chronic Fatigue Syndrome must face (CFS). Discussions on CFS frequently centre on the physical symptoms, but there can be just as many challenges to overcome in the mental maze. For someone with CFS, the mental fog they create can be just as crippling as the physical symptoms.

The core of the issue is not only the body but also the mind, where exhausting patterns and negative ideas can aggravate the clinical signs of chronic fatigue syndrome. If left unchecked, this mental spiral can worsen the sufferer's sense of wellbeing and make them feel even more exhausted all the time.

Ignoring the psychological side of chronic fatigue syndrome puts us at danger of missing a crucial part of the illness, which could result in a poorer quality of life and an insufficient recovery. However, what if there was a method to support the physical treatments for CFS by gently guiding the mind into a state of positivity and balance?

Then along comes Cognitive Behavioral Techniques (CBT), a ray of light in the frequently muddy seas of managing Chronic Fatigue Syndrome. Cognitive behavioural therapy (CBT) is a type of psychotherapy that has been empirically demonstrated to be successful in changing the way people think, which can help with a variety of psychological problems, including CFS treatment.

The first step in using CBT with CFS patients is to recognise and comprehend the negative thought patterns that are frequently associated with this condition. We then proceed to gently question and reinterpret these ideas in order to foster a more optimistic and grounded way of thinking.

Together, let's go off on this adventure. We have to first train our minds to be detectives, identifying the nagging negative thoughts that are interfering with our lives. One might mutter, "I will never get better." "I am worthless," mutters someone else. These ideas choke the bright blooms of progress and hope like weeds.

Once these are recognised, we question them. Do you really think you'll never get better? Haven't some days been better than others? Are you really useless, or is this a description you've unfairly applied to yourself when you're feeling hopeless? These are the sharp object that we use to pull out the weeds.

And thus we sow new seeds of idea. We could say, "I have good days and bad days." "I offer my own special contributions." These are the kinds of ideas that will grow into a better way of thinking—one that helps, not hurts, our journey with CFS.

Studies have demonstrated that patients who participate in cognitive-behavioral therapy frequently report improvements in both mental and physical symptoms, providing empirical support for the effectiveness of CBT in treating CFS. It's as though altering the storey in one's mind might occasionally alter how one's body reacts.

Although CBT is the mainstay of psychological psychotherapy for CFS, it is not the only way to address the issue. In an integrated approach to CFS management, other tactics like as mindfulness, graded exercise therapy, and pacing approaches are also essential. But one should never undervalue the power of the mind, and cognitive behavioural therapy (CBT) offers a methodical way to do just that.

When you include these methods into your everyday routine, the mist starts to clear. Imagine a time in the future when you feel empowered and have the resources to manage not only your body but also your mind—a future in which your thoughts become friends in your fight against CFS.

In summary, managing Chronic Fatigue Syndrome requires a multimodal strategy due to its complexity. With the help of cognitive behavioural techniques, we may effectively address and alter the thought processes that underlie the syndrome. By using these methods, we enter a new world of possibilities, one in which our thoughts are a means of returning our vitality and the mind is a doorway to healing. This, my dear reader, is simply a peek into the art of managing Chronic Fatigue Syndrome, where the secret to a life full of health and vitality is the harmony of body and mind.

Energy Allocation and Task Planning

Have you ever had a sense of being precariously balanced between the overwhelming fog of exhaustion that envelops you and the want to act? As your guide on this perilous voyage through Chronic Fatigue Syndrome (CFS), my dear reader, I will illuminate the way to efficient energy allocation and task planning—a ray of hope amidst the storm.

Think of your life as a well-composed symphony, with your daily duties acting as the harmony and your energy as the melody. Despite the difficulties posed by CFS, our ultimate goal is this peaceful state of being, in which your energy flows in perfect harmony with the beat of your everyday life.

Make sure your toolbox is ready before the first note is played. An open heart to adjust, a personal planner, and a thorough awareness of your own energy patterns are essential. These aren't just things; they're extensions of your desire to succeed.

See the bigger picture: we will map your energy landscape first, and then we will rank jobs according to how much energy they require. We will then create an adaptable daily schedule that honours your body's limitations.

1. Monitor your energy levels for a period of two weeks. Take note of the highs and lows. Do evenings speak promises of vitality, or are mornings your ally?

2. Make a to-do list every day. Mark them as necessary, crucial, or optional. Recognize that not every assignment is equal and that some can wait in the wings while others demand more attention.

3. Make a plan using the information gleaned from your task hierarchy and energy map. When you are at your busiest, schedule the more demanding acts. Intermissions are a time to rest, not to retreat, so save the troughs for that.

4. Include brief rest intervals. Consider them as the musical pauses that build to the next note. These rejuvenating breaks are powerful; they lift your soul.

Pay attention. The enemy of equilibrium is overexertion. Pay attention to the whispers in your body; they frequently indicate an approaching storm. And never forget that this symphony is all about adaptability; even though the notes fluctuate, the music never stops.

When will you know that your masterwork is finished? when the days conclude in quiet satisfaction rather than tiredness. Monitor your development. Adjust as needed. An effective plan is one that inspires accomplishment rather than exhaustion.

If you happen to strike an unharmonious note, don't give up. Evaluate and make necessary adjustments. Maybe you needed more energy to complete a task than you thought, or maybe exhaustion caught you off guard. Recalibrate the beat and adjust the scale, and the symphony will return to you.

—-

So, are you prepared to take the baton of wisdom and command the magnificent orchestra that is your life? Now let's get started and let the energy and task planning music take us to the pinnacle of productivity and well-being.

Shut your eyes for a little while. Take a deep breath and release the tension. Is there a life you can picture in which everything you do is in perfect balance with your energy reserves? a life in which you masterfully and gracefully direct the flow rather than allowing CFS to set your pace. This is our journey, my reader   to live a peaceful life that flows with the quiet rhythms of relaxation and the melodies of our strengths.

You need to gather some necessary tools before we set out on this odyssey. First, a deep understanding of your own energy oscillations, similar to being familiar with the strings of an instrument. And finally, a planner—not just any planner, but one that will serve as your daily painting canvas. Finally, a pinch of adaptability, since even the best-laid plans sometimes require a little creative licence.

Pause. Step back and look at the big picture that is your life. We must lay out the steps in order to start this energy and job management artistry. We will create a customizable daily schedule by mapping your energy, setting priorities for your chores, and balancing them. The cornerstone for our finer methods will be this wide brushstroke.

Think of your energy as a vibrant colour wheel, with each colour denoting a different intensity of strength. It's up to us to place these colours so they provide the clearest image of your life.

1. Your energy fluctuates, just like the waves in the ocean. For two weeks, watch your patterns and record the times you crest and withdraw. Our planning is based on this self-awareness.

2. Assign roles to your chores; some are lead players, requiring immediate attention, while others are ensemble members, significant but not urgent. Then there are the understudies, which are jobs that can be completed to cover for absences when energy allows.

3. Create your daily schedule using your work hierarchy and energy map as guides. During your peak periods, high-energy tasks take the lead, while during your slower periods, lower-energy jobs play supporting roles.

4. The performances themselves are not as important as the intermissions. Plan brief, rejuvenating pauses to replenish your internal reserves. Your productivity has rhythm thanks to these quiet beats.

This symphony must be conducted with attention. Excessive effort is the silent robber of peace; it breeds strife. Pay attention to your body's tiny indications. And never forget that the ability to change the tempo when necessary is what defines great artistry.

When the melody of success resonates with your symphony, how will you know? Rather of feeling empty at the end, you should feel a sense of peaceful accomplishment. Record your symphony's performance in a journal and make any adjustments. A plan that improves your well-being and recognises your achievements is where you will find validation.

If you come across a note that doesn't belong, don't give up. Examine your strategy. Maybe there was more work than you expected, or you suddenly became tired. Rearrange the rhythm, change the composition, and harmony will come back.

—-

You get better at this delicate dance of energy and tasks with each stroke of the baton. Let the symphony you lead serve as an example of your tenacity and the peaceful life that lies ahead. Let's turn the pages of "The Chronic Fatigue Syndrome Mastery Bible: Your Blueprint for Complete Chronic Fatigue Syndrome Management" together and create a life in which, despite CFS's presence in the orchestra of our health, every day is a note of success and well-being.

Relaxation and Breathing Exercises

Your Oasis of Calm

Imagine that you have a sanctuary inside of you, a calm place where Chronic Fatigue Syndrome (CFS) cannot hold you. This subsection serves as your road map to that haven, taking you through the transforming potential of breathing techniques and relaxation. I'd like to urge you to take a journey through each page that will help you reduce stress and fatigue—a voyage in which your breath will become your most valuable ally.

Your goal is to become proficient in a series of breathing and relaxation exercises intended to lessen the mental and physical toll that CFS takes. These exercises are not just workouts; they are the threads that weave your well-being together, each one enhancing your ability to remain composed and resilient.

All you need to get started is a calm area, comfy clothes, and an open mind. Although a mat or cushion can make you more comfortable, your intention and focus are what will actually work their magic.

There is a clear route ahead. Using diaphragmatic breathing as a starting point, you will learn how to develop awareness before moving on to guided visualisations and progressive muscular relaxation. Every stride you take builds the foundation of your peaceful fortress.

Together, let's revitalise your practise. The foundation is diaphragmatic breathing, sometimes known as belly breathing. With one hand on your chest and the other on your abdomen, take a comfortable seat or lie down. Feel your tummy rise as you take a deep breath with your nose and then gently release it through your mouth, feeling your belly collapse. This small yet meaningful gesture can bring about calm by lowering blood pressure and pulse rate.

As you get more skilled, picture a calm environment with every breath. Maybe a golden field, the sky painted with hopeful hues by the sun's rays. Picture worry and exhaustion vanishing into the distance with every breath out.

You are to progressively tighten and relax every muscle group, starting from your toes and working your way up to your forehead. Imagine the tension dissipating as a hue, maybe the grey of storm clouds, and leaving behind the gentle blue of a clean sky.

Recall that the quality of your practise matters more than how long it lasts. The seeds of calm can be sown in even a short while. But patience is the most important thing. Allow the rhythms to find their own natural ebb and flow; don't push yourself to breathe or tense.

Breathing too shallowly can make you more anxious. In case you feel lightheaded, stop and resume your regular breathing.

Even when you're not practising, you'll know you're on the correct track when you feel at ease. If only somewhat at first, the fog of exhaustion may clear and sleep may come more easily.

If you see that your mind is resistive or straying, compassionately bring it back to you. Every time one overcomes this usual obstacle and refocuses, it is a victory.

You are carrying the essence of breathing techniques and relaxation as you end this chapter—a ray of serenity in the turbulent sea of CFS. Recall that the ability to withstand any adversity is contained in the stillness of your breath.

Graded Exercise Therapy

A Gentle Ascent to Vitality

Just picture a mountain, if you will. Its summit, covered in a soft fog, represents the life you used to have. Many people who suffer from Chronic Fatigue Syndrome (CFS) may feel that climbing this mountain is unachievable. However, there is a route called Graded Exercise Therapy (GET), which is carefully planned and progressive and offers a promising upward trajectory.

Let's explore the life of Emily, a graphic artist of 35 years old, whose world was turned upside down by CFS. The vivid imagination that had once come easily to her was now reduced to a trickle due to unwavering fatigue. Emily's struggle was not unusual, but the way she was helped to recover—tailored by a kind team that included me—was as distinct as her fingerprints.

The main problem was Emily's crippling exhaustion, which was made worse by muscle soreness and a fog that obscured her once-clear thinking. The aim was to reawaken her vigour without fanning the flames of simmering exhaustion.

Our approach—Graded Exercise Therapy—was straightforward in theory yet had a significant effect. To establish a baseline from which to work, we started by evaluating Emily's level of activity right now. Her exercise tolerance had to be gradually increased, beginning with the mildest of motions.

The outcome was like witnessing a dormant seedling come to life. Small wins along the way, like a stroll to the mailbox, a set of stretches, or a few minutes spent on a stationary bike, characterised Emily's journey. Every stride was a victory, every step forward a reason to rejoice.

However, allow me to consider this strategy. GET has its detractors, and the treatment plan needs to be tailored to the particular needs of each patient. Instead of racing to the top, it's a methodical ascent that respects your body's cues and your mind's state of preparation. Like all of my patients, Emily's input served as our compass, directing the scope and tempo of her activities.

Emily found that visual aids like activity diaries and progress charts empowered her. Her work was turned into art by them, a visual symphony of advancement.

We are able to relate Emily's tale to the broader picture of CFS management. GET is just one component of the holistic therapy that I, Dr. Ankita Kashyap, fervently endorse. Other components include dietary advice, psychological support, and alternative therapies.

Now think about this: What tiny action may you do today that could mark the beginning of your own upward journey? Emily's storey shines like a beacon, showing others the way.

In summary, mastering Chronic Fatigue Syndrome involves more than just treating symptoms; it also entails recovering the core of one's vitality. When customised and progressed at the right rate, Graded Exercise Therapy can be a game-changer on this path. You too may muster the courage to take the initial step toward reaching the pinnacle of your own well-being, just as Emily does as she gradually climbs her mountain.

Creative Outlets for Expression

A woman who once believed she was imprisoned by the intangible bonds of chronic fatigue syndrome (CFS) dips her brush into a palette of vivid hues in the peaceful seclusion of her studio. She depicts the path of her own rehabilitation with each brushstroke in addition to painting a scene of a sunset. Let's explore the sacredness of this artistic sanctuary, where treatment is drenched in self-expression.

Introducing Emily, a 35-year-old graphic designer whose life became completely black and white due to CFS. Her symptoms—constant exhaustion, fogginess in her brain, and excruciating pain—were true. Even with the medical procedures and the family's support, Emily was still lacking a crucial component of her recovery. The difficulty? to overcome the fatigue that shadowed her every day and reclaim her excitement for life.

Emily's attendance at one of my wellness workshops, where we discussed the powerful impact that creativity can have in healing, was the turning point. We steered in the direction of an unorthodox resolution: utilising art as a means of expression and CFS therapy. Emily, a novice painter, set out on this artistic journey with hesitation but hope. It was more than just learning to paint; it was about turning her weariness into something concrete and lovely.

The strategy has several facets. It entailed establishing a regimen that was both flexible and disciplined so that Emily could work on her art without aggravating her symptoms. She was given mindfulness exercises to help her stay in the moment, which transformed painting sessions into contemplative exercises. Additionally, we included mild art therapy activities to support cognitive resilience and emotional discharge.

As Emily's advisor and mentor, With pride, I observed her metamorphosis. Her colours and brushstrokes grew more assured and vibrant with each session. The outcomes could be seen in her spirit as well as on the canvas. She said she felt more 'myself', and more vibrant than she had in years. Her perspective on life brightened, her pain became more tolerable, and her sleep improved most of all. Her general quality of life improved, her activity levels rose, and her exhaustion scores declined, all of which were supported by the statistics.

When one considers Emily's journey, it becomes clear that although art served as the medium, her restored sense of self was the real masterpiece. Though the storey is full of promise and hope, it's important to recognise that the journey towards creative therapy is quite individualised. The success of such an approach depends on customising it to the interests and energy levels of each individual. What resonates with one person may not resonate with another.

Visual aids such as Emily's before-and-after paintings are more than just works of art; they are also tangible examples of the transformative potential of artistic expression. They portray a narrative that words cannot express—one of victory against the crippling effects of CFS.

This storey of imagination and recovery is not unique. It relates to the main theme of "The Chronic Fatigue Syndrome Mastery Bible," which is the significance of holistic wellness. It serves as a reminder that although supportive therapies such as artistic expression can be the lifeblood of CFS therapy, medical treatments remain the cornerstone.

As you wrap up this chapter, think about this: Which artistic avenues have you not yet pursued? Which of your interests have been dormant, just waiting for you to give them life? Maybe you are a painter, writer, musician, or gardener waiting to channel your tiredness into something else entirely.

Emily's narrative serves as an inspiration for all CFS fighters to find their own voice. It's a call to action to create your own image of well-being, where each hue, line, and shade symbolises a step toward conquering chronic fatigue syndrome. Tell me, then, what your canvas will disclose about your path to wellbeing.

I leave you with this last pearl of knowledge, hands ready to help you and a heart full of hope: Your creative spirit is not a luxury in the art of living with CFS; rather, it is an essential component. Accept it.

Developing a Personalized Management Plan

Have you ever watched a tailor work painstakingly to create a custom garment, with each stitch serving as a reminder of the individual? This, my dear reader, is the essence of what we want to accomplish for you on your journey toward managing Chronic Fatigue Syndrome (CFS): a customised plan that fits your symptoms and life circumstances exactly.

Creating a management strategy that not only works but also speaks to the specifics of your life is our primary goal. Since CFS is not a condition that fits all patients, every therapy approach needs to be as distinct as the person it is intended for. By the time you finish reading this guidebook, you will have a map, a lighthouse to help you through the confusing waters of CFS.

Before embarking on this meticulous journey, you'll need a few tools in your kit:

- A comprehensive understanding of your CFS symptoms and their patterns.

- Insight into your daily routines, dietary habits, and existing lifestyle.

- An open mind, ready to embrace change and adapt.

- A journal or digital app to track your progress and thoughts.

- A support system, whether it be friends, family, or a support group.

- Access to a healthcare or wellness professional, should you need additional guidance.

See your management plan as a mosaic, with each tile standing for a different aspect of your life. Starting with broad strokes, we will gradually install these tiles: recognising triggers, modifying lifestyle choices, organising nutritional adjustments, incorporating self-care practises, and developing coping mechanisms.

We have to comprehend the enemy first. Note the times and situations when your symptoms come on. Is it following a certain meal? During restless nights? after times of stress? Since information is a powerful tool, it serves as the cornerstone of our military strategy.

Moving on to living, let's examine the framework of your everyday life. Tai chi and yoga are examples of gentle, healing workouts that can energise you without depleting your energy. Resetting your body's clock can be facilitated by practising good sleep hygiene, which is just as important as brushing your teeth.

Let's talk about nourishment now. What you place at the altar of your body, which is your body, matters. Sometimes all it takes is a diet high in nutritious foods, low in processed sweets and excessive caffeine. But never forget that the best guide is your body's reaction.

Self-care is necessary upkeep, not a luxury. Methods such as deep breathing exercises, meditation, or even a warm bath may be just what your tired soul needs.

Coping mechanisms are your kit's armour, to sum up. Rethinking your perspective can be achieved through cognitive behavioural strategies, and pacing—becoming aware of your body's signals before they become screams—is incredibly helpful.

Be patient; there are many mistakes along the path to mastery. Begin modestly. Even something as small as changing your bedtime can have unanticipated consequences.

A word of advice: resist the need to overindulge on your "good days." Overdoing it is not your ally; consistency is.

How can you tell if your strategy is effective? It's in the small wins: the day you wake up rested, the day you get through without any major setbacks, the night you look back on your notebook and see that there have been fewer "poor" days.

Don't give up if you realise that some tactics are ineffective or you reach a plateau. Review, adjust, and confer. Perspective from other sources can occasionally reveal avenues that are concealed from your line of sight.

Consider that you are the creator of your own map of wellbeing, and that your management plan is a dynamic document that changes with you. You have the compass to guide you through the pages of "The Chronic Fatigue Syndrome Mastery Bible: Your Blueprint for Complete Chronic Fatigue Syndrome Management." Understanding is the first step on the road to mastery, and as you go, you redefine what it means to live with CFS.

Accept the process; throughout it, you will learn how to live well despite the challenges posed by chronic fatigue syndrome. Let's start writing your mastery tale together, with hope serving as your paper and determination as your ink. This storey should be one of perseverance, personal development, and the unwavering spirit of human endurance.

Community and Advocacy

Finding Community Support

A soul by the name of Maya lived in the sleepy town of Rivendell, tucked between the peaceful river and the whispering woods. Fatigue was a persistent companion that had darkened her days ever since Chronic Fatigue Syndrome (CFS) had taken her life. But in the middle of her condition's isolation, Maya found solace in the strength of her community's support system.

Maya, the protagonist of this storey, is a lively spirit imprisoned in a sluggish body that longs for understanding and connection. The difficulty? to make her way through the lonely waters of CFS and find comfort in the arms of others who genuinely understand her plight.

Maya's adventure started when she happened upon "The Rivendell Restorers," a local support group. She was able to find others who understood her quiet language of tiredness here. The club used a variety of strategies, including buddy systems, weekly meetings, and an online forum where members could share anything from helpful tips to consolation.

The results were encouraging as the weeks stretched into months. After being alone for a while, Maya's spirit was revived by the laughs and stories she shared with her new friends. The group's internet presence flourished into a thriving hub of collaboration and attendance records skyrocketed.

As one considers this case study, the metamorphosis is something to behold. Maya's experience highlights the significant influence that community support has on people who are struggling with CFS. Not only did this support system provide a short-term respite, but it also became a vital component of her continuous management approach.

Visual aids that highlight the interdependence of the group's support system, like a colourful community tree with branches symbolising each member's contribution, could be used. This picture is a metaphor for the development and fortitude that come from having strong social roots.

This isn't just Maya's storey about Rivendell; it's a little part of a bigger storey. It serves as evidence that although CFS may play a role in our tale, it need not be the main one. These kinds of gatherings foster empathy and companionship, which are invaluable resources for managing chronic conditions.

Now ask yourself this: is there a "Rivendell Restorers" near you? Or is it possible that someone just like you has the caring hands to plant the seed of such a community?

Educating Friends and Family

People who suffer from Chronic Fatigue Syndrome frequently hear murmurs of miscommunication in their lives (CFS). Just picture, if you will, the sun setting and another day coming to an end. Sarah, a colourful person whose laugh used to fill entire rooms, is currently struggling with the imperceptible restraints of CFS. Weariness follows her around like a nagging shadow, turning the routine chores that used to be easy for her into impossible undertakings.

Sarah's family, a patchwork of devoted people, finds it difficult to understand how exhausted she is. "Why is she unable to simply persevere?" they muse in private. It is their struggle, as great as the Great Wall, and it is not only Sarah's to ascend.

The strategy used to close this understanding gap was complex. I asked Sarah's family to a number of unofficial yet educational events. Here, we told the storey of CFS and created a picture that was far more vivid than any statistic on a page could ever be. We listened, we told stories, and we gained knowledge. More than just numbers were at stake; Sarah's life was at stake.

The outcome? The collective viewpoint of a family, once obscured by misinformation, started to become apparent. The cloud of uncertainty parted, exposing a way to compassion and assistance. Sarah's father, who had always associated relaxation with laziness, developed a fresh respect for the bravery required to pay attention to one's body. Her sister, formerly sceptical but now an ally, started pushing for awareness in her own social networks.

In retrospect, there were some bumps in the road. Old views and scepticism are resilient, but knowledge and life experiences have the ability to weaken even the greatest defences. Although the graphs and figures had their use, the real insight into Sarah's family's experience with CFS came from the open discussions.

The wider storey of CFS management is reflected in this microcosm of change. Teaching friends and family is an important narrative point in the novel of healing, not just a chapter in the book of coping. The load lessens and support networks become stronger when those closest to us comprehend.

Now think about your own group, dear reader. Who might benefit from some guidance to comprehend your experience with CFS better? Could a straightforward discussion, like a stone thrown into a river, cause changes in your life?

Let us remember, as this chapter comes to an end, that empathy may be developed, one heart at a time. The interactions we have with our loved ones are as much a part of the book as the pages themselves contain the recipe for treating Chronic Fatigue Syndrome.

Gaining power over CFS is not a lonely journey. It is a journey best shared with individuals who realise that every step—no matter how small—represents a victory.

Participating in Awareness Campaigns

Imagine a world in which the act of simply waking up signifies an endless battle against a wave of tiredness rather than the start of a day full of potential and enthusiasm. For people suffering from chronic fatigue syndrome, this is their reality (CFS). However, what if this very conflict has an unrealized potential for advocacy and involvement in awareness campaigns?

Chronic fatigue syndrome is a serious health concern that is sometimes cloaked in mystery and myth. Many patients' symptoms are disregarded or misinterpreted, and they go undetected. The true issue here is not so much the illness per se, but rather the widespread ignorance that exacerbates the pain.

The ramifications of this misinformation are severe: inadequate research funding, stigma, and weak support networks. In addition to dealing with their bodily problems, patients suffer from the general lack of interest in society. Imagine the additional strain that isolation would put on already worn-out shoulders.

Still, there's a glimmer of optimism. The patients themselves, who are the ones most impacted, have the key to the answer. Patients with CFS have the opportunity to use their challenges as a catalyst for change by actively engaging in awareness efforts.

The question remains: How can someone who is already struggling with exhaustion become an advocate for this cause? Starting simple and doable is the first step. Patients can first tell their stories. Personal stories have a deeper resonance than any statistics could ever have.

Think about social media's influence: a single tweet, blog post, or Instagram storey can reach thousands, if not millions of people. For individuals whose physical endurance is diminishing, digital platforms provide an accessible stage.

Efforts can be boosted by working with already-existing CFS organisations. Although these groups frequently possess the necessary resources, their messages must come from real people.

There is a wealth of efficacious evidence. Examine previous health campaigns that have effectively utilised patient advocacy, such as the surge in support for breast cancer awareness. These days, research is constantly progressing, money is abundant, and pink ribbons are everywhere. This wasn't always the case. Many voices were needed to bring about this transformation.

What happens if using social media or public speaking becomes too difficult? Next, think about the one-on-one strategy. Talking with loved ones, friends, and even medical professionals can help to promote understanding because of the strength of human connection.

Are these the only methods that awareness may be raised? Without a doubt. One might support the cause by wearing awareness emblems, writing letters to lawmakers, or taking part in research studies.

Recall that the beauty of advocacy is that it can have an influence even when it is quiet. The smallest whisper has the power to unleash a wave of transformation.

Let's now use words to create a mental image of a society in which chronic fatigue syndrome is acknowledged, studied, and effectively treated. It's a world where people who are suffering are noticed and helped instead of being unseen warriors. This isn't simply a fantasy. That is a possibility, and it starts with you.

In summary, taking part in awareness campaigns is a powerful and purposeful journey, but it is not an easy one. I implore you to think about your special place in this movement as your guide. How are you going to start?

By working together, we can create a fabric of comprehension, empathy, and action that will serve as a monument to the resilience found even in the most trying circumstances. This is our urgent summons to action, a request to take the lead in the struggle against ignorance and for a brighter future for all CFS fighters.

Advocating for Better Research

Imagine having the sensation of having completed a marathon while you slept, every morning. Your mind is cloudy, your body hurts, and no matter how much sleep you get, the fatigue follows you around like an intractable shadow. For many people with chronic fatigue syndrome, this is their everyday life rather than a passing nightmare (CFS).

As a physician and fitness coach, I have personally witnessed the debilitating consequences of this misdiagnosed illness. Myalgic encephalomyelitis, another name for Chronic Fatigue Syndrome, is a condition that has long been cloaked in mystery. Patients who seek treatment from medical professionals sometimes encounter suspicion and mistrust. Even with its starkness, the current problem is a lack of financing and research compared to the severity of CFS.

Why is advocacy so much needed? Not the syndrome in such, but the shallow knowledge of it is the main obstacle. There is more to CFS than just fatigue. It is a multi-systemic illness that is complex and can seriously hinder an individual's functioning. Without thorough investigation, we continue to be ignorant of its causes, course, and—above all—effective treatment options.

What occurs if we ignore this challenge? The repercussions are severe: many people endure agony without an appropriate diagnosis, efficient care, or the prospect of recovery. There has been a massive loss of productivity economically. The emotional toll is immense as impacted people and their families struggle with the stigma and uncertainty surrounding CFS.

What then is doable? It's time to put out a well-thought-out lobbying plan. First and foremost, we need to advocate for more money and larger-scale research that truly acknowledges the seriousness of CFS. This entails not just more research but also better, multidisciplinary investigations that take the entire range of the illness into account.

We need to get people, medical experts, and researchers together in order to implement this. We can increase awareness of CFS and convince funding agencies and lawmakers of the importance of research by assembling coalitions. Campaigns to raise public awareness are essential to this effort, as is the backing of powerful people who can spread the word.

And what constitutes success, anyway? Think about the advancements in other once misdiagnosed disorders, including depression or multiple sclerosis. Once disregarded, they are now the focus of international discussion and get substantial research funding. The kind of activism that we now need to support for CFS marked the beginning of this transition.

While financing and research should rise, we also need to look into other options. Integrative medicine has demonstrated promise when it combines traditional treatment with supplementary therapies, lifestyle changes, and psychological support. These are areas that require our whole attention, just like biomedical research does.

Promoting improved research is morally required and goes beyond simple scientific curiosity. By increasing awareness of Chronic Fatigue Syndrome, we not only help to advance medical research but also give voice to those whose experiences have been ignored for far too long. By working together, we can end this hidden pandemic and give millions of people hope around the globe. We can make sure that CFS is an illness that can be controlled and, one day, hopefully treated with your aid, rather than a life sentence.

Navigating Healthcare Systems

Imagine setting out on a journey through a maze-like woodland, where each turn seems to be the same as the previous. This is similar to figuring out the healthcare system when dealing with Chronic Fatigue Syndrome (CFS), which is an arduous and confusing journey. I, Dr. Ankita Kashyap, am a seasoned navigator in this complex maze, and I'm here to light the way to the best care for your particular CFS journey.

The main issue we face is the complexity of healthcare systems and their frequent insensitivity to illnesses like chronic fatigue syndrome. Patients may feel disoriented and unheard due to the complexity and scepticism. Have you ever felt like a faceless statistic among all the medical data? Have you been passed around between specialists, gathering mountains of paperwork with no sense of relief? For many of the CFS soldiers, this is their reality.

It is no small task to untangle this knot; if you fail to do so, the repercussions will be severe. Misdiagnoses, untreated symptoms, and skyrocketing healthcare expenditures are just a few of the setbacks that result from the physical, emotional, and financial toll that CFS takes. The human price? Incalculable.

But there's hope, so don't be afraid. A comprehensive, patient-focused method of healthcare navigation may serve as your comfort zone's compass. Together, let's walk this journey step by step, embracing tactics designed to make sure your voice is heard and that your health comes first.

First and foremost, start speaking up for your own health. This include educating yourself on CFS, including its signs and symptoms, possible therapies, and effects on your life. Create a health dossier, which includes a detailed account of your medical background, current symptoms, and previous therapies. This dossier serves as your shield, preventing misdiagnosis and guaranteeing that every medical practitioner you come into contact with is aware of the struggles you face.

Next, establish a relationship with a primary care physician who is understanding of your situation, not merely sympathetic. This partnership is essential because they will act as your point of contact, assisting you with referral networks and standing up for your needs throughout the healthcare system. A physician who genuinely hears and comprehends? That is a valuable and uncommon jewel.

Additionally, think about the cost aspects of your care. Learn what is and isn't covered by your insurance plan and why. Here, information is power. If a therapy is not covered, raise concerns, make an appeal, and contest it. Your perseverance can be the deciding factor. Insurance may appear to be a fearsome foe, but you can frequently overcome it with persistence and patience.

Don't forget to include complementary and alternative medicine (CAM) treatments in your search. I support holistic medicine because I have seen the advantages of combining complementary and alternative medicine with mainstream therapies. These treatments, which range from meditation to acupuncture, can be the final component lacking from your CFS care plan. Although they frequently involve out-of-pocket costs, think of them as an investment in your wellbeing.

Let's now discuss realistic ways to put these answers into practise. Even when things are not urgent, make routine visits with your primary care physician. Make the most of these meetings to strengthen your bond and improve your approach to healthcare. Maintain a symptoms journal and bring it to your sessions. Graphics can help you communicate the struggles you face on a regular basis.

Proof of effectiveness? It is strewn across the narratives of many patients who have assumed control over their medical path. Their increased quality of life, the constancy of their symptoms, and—most importantly—their restored sense of control serve as the evidence.

Of course, there are other options. Some patients find comfort in sharing their stories and knowledge in support groups. Others seek assistance from patient advocates, experts in navigating the complex world of healthcare. These substitutes can add more levels of support to the strategies that have been discussed.

It is undoubtedly difficult to navigate the healthcare system when you have CFS. Nonetheless, it's a route that can result in empowerment and better health outcomes if you have the appropriate tactics and a strong ally on your side. Allow this subchapter to serve as your road map as you turn the pages of "The Chronic Fatigue Syndrome Mastery Bible," leading you from a clearing full of confusion to one that offers optimal care, understanding, and hope for the future.

Engaging With Policy Makers

Imagine a world in which the act of awakening itself signals the beginning of a never-ending battle with tiredness rather than a day full of enthusiasm. For many who suffer from Chronic Fatigue Syndrome (CFS), which is marked by extreme exhaustion as well as the frustration of being misinterpreted and frequently disregarded by the very systems designed to offer assistance and support, this is their reality. I have seen firsthand the debilitating effects of this illness and the pressing need for a paradigm change in its treatment as a physician and health and wellness coach.

The key issue is how the organisations that influence our healthcare policies identify and address CFS. Despite being common, CFS is still mysterious, frequently evading diagnosis and falling in the gaps in healthcare systems. The repercussions? People still suffer, economies suffer from missed output, and medical professionals struggle to handle the illness with insufficient protocols.

Engagement—purposeful, deliberate engagement with those who wield the pen over healthcare policy—is the cure for this ill of oversight and passivity. It is a call to action for advocates, patients, and healthcare professionals to mobilise change that changes the experience of CFS sufferers as a group and goes beyond the level of the individual.

There are two parts to the strategy: advocacy and awareness. Imagine bringing captivating stories, facts, and a change roadmap to a policymaker's office instead of a protest sign. It starts with education, making sure decision-makers understand the full scope of CFS's effects as well as that it exists. Advocacy is a useful addition to this, as it involves crafting a persuasive case for particular legislative changes that can improve the situation of people with CFS.

In order to put this into action, a coalition of interested parties, including patients, families, healthcare providers, and researchers, must first be formed and brought together by a shared goal. After that, this coalition would provide a coherent agenda—a set of precise, fact-based suggestions for changing policy. Personalizing the problem is essential; testimony and anecdotes that highlight the human cost of CFS can be powerful change agents.

Have we had any success with this strategy? There are glimpses of improvement, but the war is far from over. Take into consideration the recent actions that resulted from persistent advocacy efforts, such as the adoption of clinical guidelines and increased financing for research.

One may contend that there are other options, such organising neighbourhood campaigns or filing lawsuits to compel change. These are true, but working with legislators frequently results in more systemic and long-lasting changes. Although the journey is one that calls for endurance and patience, the results could be significant and far-reaching.

Imagine a day in the future where CFS is treated with compassion, understanding, and all-encompassing support rather than being a lifelong stigma and source of neglect. This goal can be realised, but it requires us to get up, get involved, and be change agents. Will we answer the call, that is the question? Will we be the voice that doesn't stop speaking until the sounds of advancement for CFS management reverberate through the corridors of power?

In conclusion, the CFS community must communicate with legislators; it is not only a proposal. Let us keep in mind that every discussion, gathering, and proposal we make moves us one step closer to a future in which CFS is no longer a mystery but rather a disorder that is understood and treated. Come along on this adventure with me, and together we can change the treatment landscape for Chronic Fatigue Syndrome to the benefit of everybody.

Volunteering and Giving Back

Have you ever thought about how transforming giving back can be, particularly when you are the one in need of assistance? Isn't that a strange paradox? However, this paradox contains an untapped source of healing, especially for people suffering from Chronic Fatigue Syndrome (CFS).

Living with chronic fatigue syndrome is a silent odyssey fraught with uncertainty and exhaustion. The main issue here is the persistent exhaustion that doesn't just go away after a restful night's sleep. A vicious cycle of social isolation, emotional pain, and a loss of purpose may result from this.

Imagine now what would happen if this cycle continued unbroken: a possible total disengagement from society, a decline in self-worth, and an exacerbation of depression symptoms. That is a bleak image, isn't it?

So what if I told you that despite all of this, there is a glimmer of hope? For those with CFS, volunteering and making even the tiniest of communal contributions can be an empowering answer. Spending valuable energy on other people when you're already behind may seem contradictory. Nonetheless, research indicates that giving back can set off a positive feedback loop that heightens emotions of purpose and social connectedness, both of which can lead to an enhanced sense of wellbeing.

Setting out on this journey calls for a customised strategy that honours your limits and existing energy levels. Begin modestly. It could be as easy as lending a sympathetic ear to someone who is also struggling with CFS, posting about your experiences in an internet forum, or sending a sincere letter of support to a fellow warrior.

Such projects don't have to be carried out in a big manner. Decide what you are comfortable with first. Are you able to make phone calls? Can you crochet comfort products for people with CFS or create words that inspire others? Any action has the capacity to have an impact elsewhere, regardless of its magnitude.

How do we know it works, though? Look about you and you'll find touching tales of people who, while going through their own struggles, reached out to assist others and gained newfound strength. These anecdotes provide as unofficial proof, pointing the way for all of us to follow.

Although volunteering is a wonderful option, we also need to think about other approaches for the days when we don't have as much energy. Simple deeds of kindness might be as simple as smiling at someone or providing useful materials. What matters is not the gesture's size but rather its purpose, which is what really matters.

Let's discuss the pragmatics. How can you participate in volunteer work without endangering your health? First, decide what your boundaries are and make sure the group or people you want to assist know what they are. It's important to be flexible, both for you and them. Second, choose positions that are compatible with your present skill set. For example, remote possibilities can be great because they let you participate from the comfort of your own home.

Now just pause to picture the possibilities. Can you now perceive yourself as both a compassionate provider and a recipient of compassion? This dual position has the potential to be quite powerful.

Recall that the goal is to strike a harmonious balance where your deeds of service fuel you rather than drain you, not to overextend yourself. It's about identifying the ideal place where self-care and empathy for others converge.

In conclusion, learning the skill of volunteering and giving back can open up a new depth of healing, even though Chronic Fatigue Syndrome may feel like it's draining you of your vitality. It serves as a subtle reminder that we are all valuable to the world, even in our most vulnerable moments. As you wrap up this chapter, think about one simple thing you can change today. I mean, isn't the beauty of life in the relationships we have and the help we provide one other?

Innovations in CFS Research and Treatment

Current Research Landscape

One illness that defies a comprehensive comprehension amid the maze of contemporary medical riddles is Chronic Fatigue Syndrome (CFS). The intricate pattern of symptoms associated with CFS is a challenge to both patients and medical professionals. But what if I told you that, little by little, the curtain is rising, revealing revelations that have the power to alter lives? Join us as we take a tour of the state of research today, where experts from all around the world are working nonstop to plant the seeds of hope.

The idea is straightforward: although CFS is a complex and perplexing illness, new research is pointing to potential treatment options and improved management. Previously, the storey depicted hopelessness and dead ends, but now we are starting to outline a path toward resiliency and renewal.

The growing body of knowledge regarding the biochemical foundations of chronic fatigue syndrome provides the main evidence for this encouraging change. Once believed to be solely psychological, new research has found physiological signs supporting the actual reality of CFS, including altered immune system responses and inflammatory biomarkers. These discoveries are critical because they open the door to focused therapies that go beyond treating symptoms alone.

When looking more closely, it is impossible to ignore the intriguing studies on the gut-brain axis and how it relates to CFS. New research points to a connection between the intensity of CFS symptoms and disruptions in the gut microbiome. This understanding not only helps to clarify the illness but also pave the way for cutting-edge treatments like tailored diet regimens and probiotic treatments.

But there are challenges on the way to enlightenment. Critics dispute assertions of progress by pointing to the absence of a single diagnostic standard and the variation in patient response to therapies. They contend that any alleged advancements are questionable because there isn't a clear definition.

I respond with a refutation based on the fact that CFS is a spectrum illness that affects people differently depending on who it affects. Therefore, while a universal answer may be illusive, this does not diminish the importance of tailored strategies based on thorough research. With each research study and each trial, we are assembling a puzzle that, when finished, will show a mosaic of approaches customised to each particular scenario rather than a single, universal solution.

Neurology provides more proof in favour of this theory. Another piece of the jigsaw is the latest study on neuroinflammation and its potential connection to symptoms of chronic fatigue syndrome. Furthermore, improvements in neuroimaging are starting to highlight possible structural alterations in the brains of CFS patients, which may result in breakthroughs in both diagnosis and therapy.

The conclusion, which is both strong and upbeat, is that human inventiveness and perseverance have led to the current level of CFS research. We view the world through the prism of reliable, confirmed knowledge; where there were just questions before, answers are now beginning to emerge, and where hope was once confined, it is now flourishing.

For a little moment, picture a world in which CFS is an enemy that can be defeated rather than a mysterious phantom. Imagine a healthcare system where the term "it's all in your head" is outlawed and patients receive individualised therapy that target the root cause of their pain.

How do we get to that future state? via persistent investigation, unshakable dedication, and cooperation between medical professionals, researchers, and patients. Even though the route may be lengthy and twisting, we are carving out a path back to a life that is ours.

So, dear reader, while we teeter on the edge of comprehension, I ask you to consider this: what would this entail for individuals affected by CFS? How might millions of people's lives be affected in a concrete way by these scientific discoveries? As we close this continuing storey, let us cling to the hope that knowledge breeds power: the ability to conquer CFS and give life back to people who have been yearning for it.

Let this subchapter conclude by acting as a call to action and a ray of optimism. The field of research is always changing, and our approaches to managing CFS must also change. Through "The Chronic Fatigue Syndrome Mastery Bible," we will explore the multitude of methods that encapsulate the essence of holistic medicine. Together, we will investigate how dietary adjustments, psychological counselling, lifestyle changes, and self-care practises work in concert to create a comprehensive management plan for CFS.

Understanding that each piece of data, study, and patient's storey is a thread in the healing tapestry is the first step on the path to mastery. Let's weave these threads with tenderness, empathy, and the unwavering conviction that a brighter tomorrow is ahead.

Emerging Treatments and Therapies

Every step toward innovation in the maze-like management of Chronic Fatigue Syndrome (CFS) offers hope to individuals caught in its web. Imagine living in a world where vitality is restored, life blossoms with renewed enthusiasm, and the weariness that follows you everywhere fades away. This is the goal that drives us as we look for cures and treatments that are just emerging.

Take Maya as an example. She is a graphic designer, and when CFS struck, her world went black and white. Her formerly creatively filled days turned into a series of draining obstacles. Maya faced more than simply physical exhaustion; her daily battle was exacerbated by mental fog and a lack of consensus among doctors regarding her illness.

Maya's quest for healing led her to become the focal point of an innovative study investigating a unique therapy that blended holistic wellness coaching with biophysical therapies. Her specific problem was met with a symphony of medical skill, psychological assistance, and lifestyle transformation.

It was a multifaceted strategy. Initially, a series of specific dietary supplements was prescribed to tackle any possible mitochondrial dysfunction, or a malfunction of the cell's power plant. We also started her on a mildly graded exercise programme at the same time, which was intended to raise her activity levels without making her feel exhausted afterward. The psychosocial component of CFS was addressed by using cognitive behavioural therapy and mindfulness meditation.

Despite taking time, the outcomes were impressive. Maya felt more alive, the mist started to clear, and hope came back into her eyes. Data showed that her fatigue scores had improved by 40%; while this was by no means a cure, it was a big step in the right direction toward her life being back.

By considering Maya's experience, we can gain a deeper understanding of the intricacy of CFS and the demand for individualised treatment programmes. Although the slower rate of advancement and the necessity for more empirical support may give rise to criticism, the actions made here are transformative seeds that could yield a healing harvest.

If Maya's energy levels were represented on a graph, the increasing slope would represent her renewed enthusiasm for life. This graphic help may act as evidence of the promise that new treatments hold.

Maya's narrative represents just a small portion of the overall picture of CFS care. It relates to the main idea of this book, which is a thorough blueprint that incorporates both modern science and conventional wisdom. We are at the cusp of a new era in which a patchwork of hope is provided by newly developed treatments and therapies.

What about people who are still looking for their big break through, though? But what about all the other people who, like Maya, wish they could go back to being their colourful selves?

The range of CFS symptoms is reflected in the variety of emerging medicines and treatments. The field is constantly changing, ranging from immunomodulatory treatments that aim to correct immune system malfunctions to the innovative use of antiviral drugs that target underlying illnesses. Biotechnology and genomics developments are opening the door to personalised medicine strategies that have the potential to completely transform CFS treatment.

We also cannot undervalue the influence of the mind-body link. Evidence supporting the benefits of integrative therapies like acupressure, yoga, and Tai Chi in the management of chronic conditions is driving their popularity. New opportunities arise even in the field of digital health interventions, where self-management and symptom tracking are supported by applications and web programmes.

It is crucial that we take a balanced approach as we navigate these waters. For some people, a given treatment might not be the catalyst for a comeback. This is the complex puzzle that is CFS, and every piece needs to be placed carefully and precisely.

I am here to support you at the forefront of your journey as a health and wellness coach. My team of interdisciplinary professionals and I are committed to creating a path that is as distinct as the person taking it. By implementing dietary adjustments, self-care practises, and lifestyle adjustments, we provide a solid basis for these new treatments.

Even yet, we need to question ourselves, "Are we ready to welcome the changing tides?" as we look into this bright future. How can we guarantee that these innovations are available to every person with CFS?

So, as we come to an end of this subchapter, dear reader, let me leave you with one last thing to consider: Where might your thread fit within the overall picture of managing CFS and the evolving healing pattern?

Genetics and Personalized Medicine

Imagine a future in which your individual health riddle could be solved by a straightforward DNA test. This is not some far-off future; rather, it is the rapidly emerging field of customised medicine, which has the potential to significantly improve the lives of those suffering from chronic fatigue syndrome (CFS).

Let me, Dr. Ankita Kashyap, take you on a captivating journey through a scenario in which tailored medicine and genetics come together to tackle the mystery of CFS.

Introduce yourself to Maya, a lively graphic designer whose life took an unexpected turn when exhaustion wrapped itself around her. Raj, an entrepreneur whose boundless energy seemed to vanish over night, was also perplexed. distinct life, same predicament.

The main obstacle they faced was the elusive nature of chronic fatigue syndrome (CFS), which is marked by extreme fatigue that is not relieved by rest and is made worse by mental or physical exertion. Not only were the symptoms problematic, but there was no definitive diagnostic procedure or one-size-fits-all course of treatment.

Our method was novel. We explored the realm of genetics, where our secrets about health are whispered in our DNA. We tried to identify the variants that might be related to their CFS through specialised genetic testing.

The outcomes had a revolutionary effect. While Raj's genetic profile indicated abnormalities impacting his cellular energy metabolism, Maya's demonstrated a tendency toward specific immunological dysfunctions. Equipped with this understanding, tailored treatment plans were developed. While Raj's approach concentrated on mitochondrial health and metabolic support, Maya's plan placed more emphasis on immunological regulation.

The result? Profound. Maya saw a dramatic decrease in her inflammatory symptoms. Raj stated that his energy and cognitive abilities have increased. Their experiences serve as examples of how customised medicine can be used to treat CFS.

We learn from this trip through genetics and customised medication that CFS is not an unbeatable opponent. The knowledge acquired highlights the significance of a customised strategy and acknowledges that a patient's genetic composition can provide insight into their path to wellbeing.

Imagine two charts: one active and illuminating Raj's metabolic pathways, and the other bright and detailed, charting Maya's genes connected to immunity. These visual aids function as symbols of optimism and uniqueness in addition to being scientific exhibitions.

This storey represents a small portion of the enormous potential that genetics and customised medicine provide for the treatment of CFS. In order to customise a health blueprint for each individual that is as distinct as their DNA, it is necessary to understand them at the most basic level.

What about you, though? Have you given any thought to the potential that is still unrealized within your genetic code? Is it the component that's missing from your puzzle of vigour and vitality?

As we get to the end of this chapter, I would like you to consider what individualised care plans and genetic insights might be able to give you in your journey with CFS. This is a call to rethink how we see and address this complicated syndrome—not the end. Rather, it is a fresh start. The future is yours to grasp; it is hopeful, personalised, and awaits you.

Recall that you are more than just a case, a number, or an enigma in the realm of chronic fatigue syndrome. Being a singular person, you possess a tale imprinted in your very cells, ready to be read and comprehended in order to lead you to your own personal fulfilment.

Let us step boldly into that future, together.

The Role of Technology in Management

Technology appears as a ray of hope in the complicated process of managing Chronic Fatigue Syndrome (CFS); when used properly, it can show the way to improved health and wellbeing. Consider Emma's tale: she was a bright graphic designer before CFS cast a shadow on her life. The array of symptoms was relentless, the exhaustion unwavering, and the fog in my head thick. Emma's storey is a note in the symphony of CFS stories, not a stand-alone storey.

The tools that changed Emma's approach to managing her CFS are also important characters in her storey, in addition to her medical professionals. Despite being silicon-based, these unsung heroes played a crucial role in her quest to restore her energy.

Emma's battle was primarily about three challenges: keeping track of her treatment schedule, regulating her energy levels, and dealing with the erratic symptoms of CFS. These activities were too difficult for her to handle alone, and conventional approaches were unable to give her the assistance she required.

Now for the Approach or Solution: a collection of gadgets and apps that have been carefully chosen and are meant to fit in perfectly with Emma's life. With a few taps on a symptom tracker app, she could easily note changes in her condition, which became her daily confidant. Her activity levels were tracked by a wearable gadget, which alerted her when it was time to take a nap. Her diet was customised with the use of specialised meal-planning software to increase her energy. With the use of a sleep tracker, even her sleep—that elusive restorer—was able to settle into a calming regularity.

The effects took some time to manifest, but they were significant. Emma gained clarity on previously unknown aspects of her health. As patterns developed, it became easier to identify her triggers and the solutions that helped her feel better. Her symptom tracker data eventually showed a link between stress and flare-ups, which inspired her to start including mindfulness exercises in her daily routine.

Upon analysing and reflecting on Emma's experience, it becomes evident that technology served as both a companion and a catalyst for transformation, rather than a cure-all. There were difficulties, such as the early learning curve, the requirement for constant participation, and the sporadic technological difficulties. However, there was no denying the empowerment it promoted.

Visual aids, such as the graphs and charts produced by Emma's applications, let her care team precisely adjust their approach by turning her subjective experiences into objective statistics.

This example relates to the broader storey about how technology may be used to manage CFS and shows that it can be a powerful tool in our fight to understand this mysterious illness. It provides a peek at a day where healthcare and technology are closely intertwined and each person has a customised wellness path.

And now for you, dear reader, a Transition Thought or Question: How may technology affect the way you personally oversee CFS? Is it the piece that's been missing from your puzzle, the secret to becoming a more colourful version of yourself?

Let's remember the power of simplicity as we continue this exploration. The biggest change is frequently brought about by using the simplest instrument consistently and consciously; complex solutions are not always the answer. Listen to your body's rhythm and allow technology to magnify it.

In conclusion, technology plays a revolutionary—rather than merely supplemental—role in the management of chronic fatigue syndrome. It marks the beginning of a new age in personalised medicine, where more sophisticated understandings of each individual's distinct experience with CFS are made possible by data-driven decision-making. Let's embrace these digital friends as we move forward because they offer the possibility of a happier, more active tomorrow.

Clinical Trials and How to Participate

Imagine a society in which the mystery behind Chronic Fatigue Syndrome (CFS) is not only comprehended but also successfully treated. where every victory moves us one step closer to freeing people from the grip of never-ending fatigue. Allow me to now lead you into a world of possibilities where your involvement may spark ground-breaking discoveries.

Think of 35-year-old Sarah, a graphic designer whose vivid inventiveness was masked by the lingering fog of CFS. Beside her is Dr. Ravi Patel, an industrious investigator committed to deciphering the intricacies of this ailment. Collectively, they embody the essence of a clinical trial - a ray of hope amidst the disorder caused by chronic illness.

The obstacle in their path? to assess the effectiveness of a novel dietary intervention designed to reduce CFS symptoms. Like many others, Sarah had stumbled through a maze of therapies with little time for recovery. On the other hand, Dr. Patel's method was distinct. It was based on the complementary principles of holistic health and nutritional science, reflecting the values we uphold in our work.

The approach was twofold: first, a diet plan full of nutrient-dense foods was carefully designed to lower inflammation and boost mitochondrial function. The trial's goal was to nurture the full individual, not only test a hypothesis, with lifestyle adjustments and a strong support network in place.

The results started to show promise as the weeks became into months. Sarah's energy levels increased noticeably, and her "brain fog" started to lift. Even though the results was preliminary, it was encouraging—a glimmer of light amid the thick cloud of CFS research.

When considering this instance, more insights are revealed than just the data. They emphasise how important individualised treatment is for managing CFS and how effective dietary changes can be. However, they also subtly warn against drawing haste because a single study is simply a small part of the enormous body of scientific knowledge.

Although they are not included here, visual aids might help explain Sarah's and others' life-changing experiences. Charts showing increased energy levels and graphs showing enhanced cognitive function are examples of hope.

Let's now extend this vignette to encompass the larger field of clinical trials. As someone navigating the rough seas of CFS, how can you participate in such groundbreaking research?

Enrolling in a clinical trial is an adventure unto itself. It starts with comprehension, which entails learning about the goals, methods, and possible implications of the research. A nexus of information is provided by resources like clinicaltrials.gov, which lists trials that are actively looking for volunteers. Additionally, your healthcare professional can act as a beacon of hope, directing you toward trials that complement your particular medical path.

Eligibility is the next step after you've found a trial that appeals to you. To guarantee both the integrity of the data and the safety of participants, clinical studies have rigorous eligibility requirements. You are in a partnership with the study team, so interact with them, raise any questions you may have, and remember that your health comes first.

If the stars align and you qualify, get ready for an adventure filled with exploration and hard work. A commitment to transparency, frequent check-ins with the study team, and adherence to particular protocols are frequently necessary for participation.

However, why take on this adventure? Aside from the appeal of adding to the body of knowledge in medicine, taking part in clinical trials provides a distinct chance to receive state-of-the-art care from a team of health-focused specialists.

To pique your interest, allow me to ask you this: Could your involvement be the secret that opens new avenues for CFS management?

As we come to the end of this subchapter, remember Sarah's tale and the potential of clinical trials. Involvement contributes to a shared goal of learning and healing rather than merely being an act of bravery on an individual basis.

I encourage you to think, to investigate, and maybe even to take the initial step toward joining a storey that goes beyond the self—a storey of optimism, advancement, and the unwavering quest of health.

Let the idea of your possible part in this enormous project serve as the spark that propels you through the next chapters as you turn the page. Because not only do these pages contain knowledge, but they also have the ability to change lives, including your own.

Global Collaborations and Efforts

Envision a world in which intangible strands entwine the knowledge of innumerable people to achieve a single objective, connecting every region of the earth. This serves as the setting for our narrative, which combines the powerful force of international cooperation with the overwhelming complexity of chronic fatigue syndrome (CFS).

Here come the major players: a group of scientists, physicians, and patient advocacy organisations with a variety of backgrounds in science and culture. These people are the leaders in the unwavering quest to comprehend and treat CFS, both inside the prestigious halls of academia and on the front lines of clinical practise.

The main obstacle? CFS is a mystery, a chameleon of a disease that defies easy classification and is resistant to standard care. People all over the world experience excruciating pain, exhaustion, and a plethora of other symptoms; frequently, they feel misunderstood and ignored by the very medical community they seek assistance from.

Our approach had many facets, just like the situation was complicated. Our approach involved combining state-of-the-art research, patient-centered care approaches, and cutting-edge technology to create a comprehensive set of solutions specifically designed to address this complex illness.

What were the outcomes? Improved patient outcomes resulted from the integration of traditional medicine with biopsychosocial techniques in Norwegian clinics. Unprecedented insights were gained in the United States through the application of big data analytics, which revealed patterns in patient symptoms and treatment responses. Additionally, in Australia, telemedicine programmes have bridged gaps caused by long-standing geographic limitations to provide professional treatment to even the most isolated patients.

But let's take a moment to think. Every win has a lesson to be learned. The biopsychosocial model was criticised for oversimplifying the biological basis of CFS. The method was not without its detractors. However, every obstacle we faced strengthened our commitment as a team and encouraged more creativity.

We demonstrated the scope and influence of our joint efforts with visual aids like patient improvement statistics graphs and worldwide maps with CFS research hotspots highlighted. They acted as an example of what happens when people around the world band together for health.

This case study, which is a microcosm of the greater storey, emphasises how crucial international cooperation is to the fight against CFS. Our collective expertise and life lessons serve as our armour against this cunning foe.

Now think about this: What if the secret to solving the puzzles surrounding CFS is not found in a single laboratory, but rather in the interstice, in the language that unites us all in our global conversation?

By changing up the tempo of our scientific investigation, we discover creativity in unison and strength in diversity. The ties of cooperation link us together across borders, uniting us in our humanity and our vision of a future unencumbered by Chronic Fatigue Syndrome.

We delve deeper into the ocean of group efforts and emerge with pearls of knowledge, wellness methods, and hope for those affected by chronic fatigue syndrome within the pages of "The Chronic Fatigue Syndrome Mastery Bible: Your Blueprint for Complete Chronic Fatigue Syndrome Management."

Could you, the reader, be the one to pen the next chapter in our worldwide storey, spurred on to join the ranks of those who dare to dream of a world in which CFS is but a memory? Think of the strength of togetherness, and let's march forward as a group because the melody of healing is most audible in the harmony of our voices.

We therefore end this chapter with an ellipsis rather than a full stop—an invitation to carry on the discussion, to build on the work of those who came before us, and to pave the way for a time when Chronic Fatigue Syndrome is understood and treated rather than just tolerated.

Customizing Your CFS Management Plan

Assessing Your Symptom Profile

For a brief period, picture your body as a well-tuned orchestra, with each instrument playing a part in the overall harmony of wellbeing. However, the entire melody falters when one instrument goes out of tune. This discordance is similar to Chronic Fatigue Syndrome (CFS), a confusing illness that throws off life's rhythms. The first step in learning how to effectively manage chronic fatigue syndrome (CFS) is to carefully evaluate and map out our symptom profile.

Making a thorough map of your symptoms is the obvious goal here, as it will be a vital tool in navigating the complexity of CFS. This map will not only help us comprehend how your ailment presents uniquely, but it will also show us the way to individualised management plans that are in line with your body's and mind's particular requirements.

Let's set up our tools before delving into the nuances of symptom evaluation. You will want a dependable pen or keyboard, a notebook or a digital app for keeping track of your symptoms, and a dedication to consistent self-reflection. With these basic tools, we are ready to go out on our journey towards self-awareness.

The procedure of evaluating your symptom profile seems simple enough at first. It entails tracking, documenting, and evaluating your symptoms over time. However, don't let its apparent simplicity fool you—this is a deep exercise in awareness and self-discovery.

1. :
Start by impartially examining your mind and body. Let's tackle this with the inquisitiveness of a scientist investigating an intriguing occurrence. Which symptoms stand out the most? How do they fluctuate during the course of the day? Which stimuli appear to make them worse? Do trends develop over time?

2. :

Take some time throughout your day's quiet moments to write down your observations. Here, specificity is your friend. Take note of each symptom's severity, frequency, and duration. Recall that every nuance of your body in this space is worthy of being captured on camera.

3. :

Analyze the data with the precision of an artisan after several weeks of data collection. Look for causes and relationships. Which pursuits cause weariness to intensify? Exist any lifestyle decisions that appear to lessen the symptoms?

Take these mild suggestions into consideration while you record your symptoms. First, equilibrium is essential. Steer clear of the trap of excessive tracking, which can make things worse. Secondly, pay attention to your body's whispers before they become shouts; CFS can be effectively managed by early pattern recognition.

If you map your symptoms successfully, how will you know? You will experience a feeling of clarity and an awareness of your condition that is as personal as a well held secret. Your journal will provide you a complete picture of your CFS and a window into your everyday life.

If you are having trouble identifying patterns or are feeling overwhelmed by the variety of symptoms, don't give up. This is a typical thread in the intricate fabric of CFS. Consult medical experts or CFS support groups for assistance. A new set of eyes may occasionally notice a pattern that is hidden from view.

By being aware of the nuances in our symptoms, we prepare ourselves to become experts in managing Chronic Fatigue Syndrome. This first note of self-evaluation will take you to the more profound reaches of customised management, where every tactic is a purposefully chosen note that adds to the harmony of your reestablished health.

As we come to the end of this subchapter, keep in mind that evaluating your symptom profile is a continuous process that involves talking to your body. It is the foundation that supports your mastery of CFS. You create a life that hums with the song of health and vigour as you get more tuned in to the distinct rhythms of your body's requirements with every day and entry.

Setting Realistic Goals

Stepping into the Sunlight: Setting Realistic Goals

Have you ever felt as though the most basic of activities loomed like mountains, locked in the shadows? Should Chronic Fatigue Syndrome (CFS) be the darkness that envelops your potential, let's discuss strategies for bringing in the light. The road to controlling CFS is a journey of measured steps, each done with caution and purpose; it is not a sprint. The skill of realistic goal-setting is one such step.

Imagine living a life where every day seems like an overwhelming obstacle. The main problem here is not so much the weariness that clings to one like an obstinate mist as it is the innate yearning to take one's life back from its clutches. This is how many people with CFS feel. The repercussions? Overambition followed by eventual burnout that makes the symptoms worse in a vicious cycle.

What if I told you there was a way to get out of this now? Setting reasonable yet attainable goals is the deceptively simple solution. This is about aligning your sights with the boundaries of your present talents, not about lowering them.

The first step in implementation is to comprehend your own physique. Start every day by thinking back. What can you do today with ease? Write it down. Maybe it's only a quick stroll, an hour at work, or maybe simply a chat with a buddy. Greater successes are paved with smaller victories.

The tales, in addition to the science, provide evidence of the effectiveness of this method. I've witnessed patients change their life by adopting this concept. They began with the fundamentals and progressively increased their ability, discovering that as time went on, their perspectives grew wider.

It is accurate to say that there are other options. While some advise taking a more passive stance and waiting for the good days to arrive, others advise pushing through the exhaustion. However, in my experience, taking the middle route frequently results in the finest outcomes. It involves identifying boundaries and persistently but gently pushing them in that direction rather than using force.

Picture the sun rising and warming the world with its rays. Each ray is an objective you have set for yourself, one that is doable and illuminates the shadowy areas of CFS. Recall that dawn arrives gradually rather than all at once. Your recuperation will also progress, one doable objective at a time.

"A journey of a thousand miles begins with a single step," as Lao Tzu once said. Should we proceed in that manner jointly?

Incorporating Flexibility Into Plans

It's like sailing the high seas; the winds and waves might change course at any time when you're navigating the maze that is Chronic Fatigue Syndrome (CFS). As an experienced holistic health captain, I have seen firsthand the turbulent waves that people with CFS have to ride. Although the journey is difficult for the faint of heart, you can steer toward calmer waters if you have the correct compass.

If you will, picture a strategy that is so inflexible that it breaks with the smallest hint of modification. This is the situation that many people with CFS encounter. The main problem with this ailment is its changeable nature; symptoms can vary in severity, frequency, and length. What is beneficial one day can not be the next, and this volatility can make a strict management plan not only useless but, in certain situations, harmful to an individual's health as well.

Plans that are not flexible have many negative effects. When objectives are not reached, they may result in feelings of dissatisfaction and failure. They may make symptoms worse by pressuring a person to follow a routine for which their body isn't ready on any given day. This can therefore result in a physically and psychologically taxing cycle of aggravation and recuperation.

Thus, adding flexibility to our management strategies' design is the answer. A flexible strategy enables modifications based on daily symptom assessment and allows for adaptation to the constantly shifting tides of CFS. This is not to imply that buildings should be abandoned; quite the contrary. Instead, the goal is to create a strategy that is both supporting and flexible by incorporating flexibility like a golden thread into the framework.

The first step in putting such a plan into practise is realising how unpredictable CFS may be. From there, we establish general objectives that allow for a variety of activities that may be adjusted based on an individual's daily capabilities. If exercise is included in the plan, we may do anything from a moderate walk to a more strenuous workout, based on each person's daily energy levels.

The testimonials of those who have followed this path provide evidence of the effectiveness of this technique. Patients frequently report feeling more in control of their condition and experiencing less stress and worry as a result of managing it. They achieve a balance between activity and rest, which is essential for controlling chronic fatigue syndrome, by paying attention to their body and modifying their plans accordingly.

Other tactics are also worth mentioning, even if this adaptable framework is essential. Careful planning with backup plans for the worst days of the future brings comfort to some. Some adopt a more intuitive stance, allowing their body's cues to direct their actions. Every approach has advantages and can be customised to meet the requirements and tastes of the individual.

Recall that the choices are infinite and the horizon is wide as you navigate these waters. By being adaptable, you create a personalised plan that takes into account the ups and downs of your journey with CFS. This is a calculated move that gives you the ability to face the obstacles ahead of you with grace and resiliency rather than a surrender to the condition.

Shall we pause for a moment to consider this? How many times do we stick to our plans because we think that straying from them would cause chaos? But isn't adaptation and change fundamental to life itself? By creating a flexible plan, we become architects of our own well-being, constructing a structure that flexes but does not break under the weight of uncertainty, freeing us from the whims of the unpredictable.

Think about the strength of one flexible thought: "Today, I will do what I can, and that is enough." Use this as your compass while you navigate the erratic path of CFS. Healing waters flow most easily in this area of self-compassion and adaptation.

Finally, I would like to extend an invitation to you, my dear reader, to learn the art of flexibility in managing chronic fatigue syndrome. It is an invaluable instrument that offers optimism in the frequently gloomy waters of this ailment. With it, you may design a path that is exclusively your own, one that respects the knowledge of your body and takes into account the subtleties of your experience. This is just one part of your lifelong learning process to become a CFS expert; it goes much beyond what can be found in a book.

As you sail the oceans of CFS with flexibility as your dependable ally, may your sails be full and your compass true. Together, one flexible strategy at a time, we map out the path to wellbeing.

Regular Review and Adjustment

Just as the sun rises, promising a fresh day, so too should our approach to managing Chronic Fatigue Syndrome (CFS) be flexible enough to accommodate new ideas and modifications. It's a journey, frequently one in which we must negotiate the erratic seas of our own bodies' reactions.

Have you ever thought about how our everyday routines and our bodies interact in such a complex way? The silent cues that something needs to change? These signals form the basis of our current discussion. It is critical for people with CFS to understand when a management plan needs to be reviewed and gently pushed in a different direction.

Imagine that you've created a detailed plan that is a symphony of food selections, sleep schedules, and workout routines that are all in sync with the distinct rhythm of your body. It has served as a ray of hope and a compass in the haze of exhaustion. What transpires, then, if the notes stop resonating and the music begins to falter?

This is the main obstacle we face. A CFS management plan that is not regularly reviewed and adjusted risks becoming as outdated as a map of an ancient city, missing many of its current streets and alleys. What is the outcome? a route that makes one feel more exhausted, frustrated, and like they're lost on their own health journey.

What then is the way to keep your CFS management strategy current and functional? The key is realising the value of routine reviews, which are methodical assessments that guarantee your plan changes as you do.

Let's explore the actions required to maintain your management plan as lively and active as life itself.

First, plan a review period. Set aside specific days in your calendar as milestones, whether they be quarterly or bi-monthly.

Throughout these assessments, consider where you are right now: Do your symptoms seem to be getting better or are they coming back stronger than before? Does your energy seem to be constant or is it erratic like a light blown by the wind?

Next, take a critical look at every element of your plan. Nutrition: Do your meals still provide you with enough energy, or do they make you feel exhausted? Exercise: does it empower you or does it deplete the reserves you've worked so hard to accumulate? Do the sheets remind you of a sleepless night, or are you waking up feeling rejuvenated?

By posing these insightful queries, you start to sketch out potential changes that might be required. Maybe you might start including more nutrient-dense foods in your diet, or maybe you should switch up your low-impact workout routine to something more suitable for your current condition. To encourage deeper sleep, it can even be as easy as making little adjustments to your sleep hygiene routine.

The numerous testimonials from others who have gone before you provide proof of the efficacy of this customised strategy. Consider Sarah, one of my patients, who saw a notable decrease in her joint discomfort and a boost in energy following dietary modifications that included more anti-inflammatory items.

Even while frequent evaluation and modification form the basis of our approach, let's not overlook the existence of other options. It has been demonstrated that mind-body practises like yoga, tai chi, and meditation not only reduce stress but may also help with CFS symptoms.

It is crucial to stay adaptable, pay attention to your body's tiny indications, and be prepared to alter the choreography as necessary when performing this dance with CFS. Recall that maintaining a constant discussion with your health is more important than adhering to a set strategy.

I'll leave you with this thought to chew over as we get closer to the finish of this chapter: When was the last time you paid attention to what your body was telling you and changed your course accordingly? Your management plan is a living document that demonstrates your flexibility and resiliency. It is not set in stone.

Finally, I implore you to approach the process of routine evaluation and modification with the same bravery and tenacity that you have demonstrated throughout your CFS journey. You might be able to master Chronic Fatigue Syndrome and not simply manage it if you are flexible and prepared to change.

Keep in mind that your health is a novel that is constantly being written; make sure that every chapter honours the dynamic storey of your life.

Working With Healthcare Professionals

There is a great sense of expectation as the sun peeks through the curtains of a calm examination room. Dr. Ankita Kashyap is sitting across from me, and the patient is tired but hopeful. Managing Chronic Fatigue Syndrome (CFS) is a journey as complex as the human body's tapestry, and in these walls we set out on a cooperative endeavour. With our combined skills, my team and I are prepared to create a management plan that is as special as the person in front of us.

Consider, for example, Maya, a middle-aged woman. She works as a librarian and enjoys reading, but the constant exhaustion and unwavering symptoms of CFS have interrupted her own storey. Our task is not limited to treating her symptoms; it is also creating a life that she can live, enjoy, and that has meaning, something that has escaped her grasp like sand grains.

Like all of our patients, Maya is the subject of a holistic approach from us. We explore lifestyle changes, looking closely at everyday habits from the perspective of wellness and carefully examining food and diet to provide her body with fuel without overtaxing it. We study psychology and counselling because we know that the body and mind are intertwined and that treating one benefits the other. Our toolkit of self-care practises includes everything from the focused, contemplative yoga to the focused, intense cognitive behavioural therapy.

The outcomes are quite telling. Maya, who was before a prisoner to her illness, now claims that her level of exhaustion has decreased by 40%. It's not a cure, but it's a big start in the right direction bringing her life back. Despite being personal, the data shows a general upward trend in success and hope. Equipped with customised treatment programmes, our patients frequently discover themselves retracing their steps to a life they thought was lost.

Upon thought, there are certain hazards on the trip. Every patient reacts differently, so what calms one person may agitate another. This is the messy, wonderful, and very human art and science of healthcare. We keep moving forward, learning and adapting along the way.

In our clinic, visual aids such as stress management diagrams and nutritional charts serve as a beacon for patients like Maya, helping them navigate the mists of chronic fatigue syndrome. These are not just educational resources; they are lifelines.

Maya's narrative is just one small part of the overall picture of CFS care. It serves as an example of the vital role that medical professionals play in creating a strategy that takes the full person—mind, body, and spirit—into account. As partners in the dance of wellbeing, where each step is expertly choreographed to the distinct beat of the individual's demands, we play the role of guide rather than dictator.

What about you, though, my dear reader? How might this storey of cooperation and individualised treatment change the way you personally experience CFS? Have you given any thought to the harmonious support system that is waiting for you under the supervision of a committed medical team?

To underline in just one sentence: You're not by yourself.

Our motto is simplicity, and we try to demystify the complexity of CFS in the language we use. We cordially invite you to accompany us on a journey of empowerment and education, as we provide enlightening but manageable explanations.

Pay attention to the rhythm of our talks, the ebb and flow of our advise, and the crescendo of hope that grows with every little accomplishment. Our conversation is a call and response with you at its centre, not a monologue.

We pepper our advice with thought-provoking quotes and illuminating conversations. As Virgil famously observed, "Health is the greatest riches," and it is through these exchanges that development is made possible.

As we come to the end of this subchapter, we go full circle to the main focus of this mastery bible, which is the thorough and all-encompassing management of chronic fatigue syndrome. Maya's storey is just a taste of what's in store for you—a testimonial to the effectiveness of individualised care.

So as you close this chapter, here's an idea to chew over as you turn the page: How may your own path to wellness unfold, working hand in hand with those who are aware of the fine balance involved in managing CFS?

Step forward, dear reader, and let us uncover that path together.

Involving Family and Friends

The world can appear to be moving slowly in the stillness of a life altered by Chronic Fatigue Syndrome (CFS), a silent movie that only you are not in control of. The importance of a network—a circle of support—becomes evident in these times of solitude, just like the sunrise does every day.

Have you ever thought about how powerful a role your loved ones can have in helping you manage CFS? Maybe it's an idea that hovers at the edge of your consciousness, an unknown place that beckons with mixed feelings of hope and trepidation.

The problem, which is frequently unsaid but profoundly felt, is that chronic fatigue syndrome is a complicated mystery. It makes weariness a part of who you are, a weariness that few people can relate to and that many misunderstand. The issue at hand is how to explain to loved ones and friends the unrelenting grip of CFS. How can you turn them from being spectators to allies in your journey?

If neglected, this gap creates a mixture of miscommunication and isolation. With good intentions but limited understanding, your loved ones could give you well-meaning counsel that doesn't meet your needs or, worse, unintentionally adds to your load.

Imagine a different situation where your inner circle actively supports your quest to wellness and recognises the seriousness of what you've gone through. This vision is stronger because of the concrete actions we can do to make it a reality rather than because of wishful thinking.

Education is the first step towards a solution. Educating others about CFS helps you move from empathy to action. Talks are the first step; sincere, open discussions that help close the gap between your reality and their perceptions.

Imagine having a nice cup of tea when you sit down with your family and tell them about your experience living with CFS in addition to the medical details. Even for a brief while, they are forced to experience the world through your eyes because of how vividly and minutely you depict it.

Furthermore, friends—those partners selected by heart rather than bloodline—can serve as your ally, confidante, and fellow helper when dealing with day-to-day challenges. Give them information on how CFS impacts you, and observe how they take initiative in both large and small ways.

How do we implement this plan? Start with books, articles, and pamphlets that provide an accurate description of CFS. After this, have a family meeting, which should be more of a conversation than a lecture. Inquire about their opinions, their worries, and whether they would be open to joining your support network.

Urge them to join you for therapy sessions or doctor's appointments. Their presence is instructive as well as consoling. They become aware of the subtleties of your illness and are better equipped to assist you.

This method is supported by more than just anecdotal evidence. Research indicates that individuals with robust social support typically experience improved health outcomes. This translates into a higher quality of life rather than just fewer hospital stays or prescription drug usage. It's important to thrive rather than just get by.

What happens if the people closest to you show resistance, lack knowledge on how to assist, or, in the worst situations, deny the seriousness of your illness? Here's where other approaches become relevant. Online and in-person support groups can provide something close to the kind of family support you so much need. They can remind you that you are not travelling alone, fill in the blanks, and give you a sense of community.

Including your friends and family in your CFS care plan is a continuous process rather than a one-time occurrence. It calls for tolerance, comprehension, and most importantly, dialogue. Even though your connections come and go, every discussion you have and every experience you share puts one more stone in the path of understanding.

It's a worthwhile route to go because, as the saying in Africa goes, "Go alone if you want to move quickly. Go together if you wish to succeed." The road with CFS is definitely a marathon rather than a sprint. And how better to navigate it than with a group of allies by your side, their combined strength resonating with every stride you take?

As we get to the end of this chapter, dear reader, let's consider the strength of unity. Recall that including your loved ones is a brave step toward holistic wellbeing rather than a show of weakness. With the appropriate strategy, your loved ones can go from being bystanders to being essential players in the storey of your health.

Let this chapter serve as a springboard for change, one that starts with a straightforward discussion, mutual comprehension, and a unified front against the epidemic of chronic fatigue syndrome. You are more powerful when you work together. Together, you can create a narrative of resiliency, optimism, and—most importantly—overcoming CFS.

Documenting Your Journey

The road to becoming an expert in Chronic Fatigue Syndrome (CFS) is frequently convoluted and cloaked in ambiguity. I urge you to chart your journey as I lead you through this maze, not only to show you the route but also to consider the distance you've covered, the challenges you've overcome, and the successes you've had. Let's explore the discipline of recording your CFS journey, which is just as important as any therapy or treatment.

You may wonder why the seemingly simple process of documentation is so important. There are several factors at play, and their importance cannot be emphasised. We'll lay out a list of these reasons here, each of which is a lighthouse that can help you gain deep self-awareness and improve the way your illness is managed.

1. Tracking Symptoms and Triggers
2. Monitoring Progress and Setbacks
3. Enhancing Communication with Healthcare Providers
4. Facilitating Emotional Release
5. Empowering Self-Advocacy

Like the tides, the ebb and flow of CFS symptoms can be unexpected. By maintaining an extensive journal, you take on the role of the health's mapper, identifying trends and subtleties that you may miss otherwise.

You'll start to see the tides as you record your daily experiences—how particular foods, activities, or even emotions might affect your symptoms. This information gives you the ability to foresee and, to the greatest extent feasible, avoid the situations that worsen your illness.

I've heard from countless people about how this straightforward exercise has changed their life. It was like "putting on a spotlight in a dark room," according to one who revealed the unseen causes of her outbursts.

Think about being able to schedule your days ahead of time, knowing that a specific stressor will probably cause you to become exhausted. This is what tracking symptoms and triggers can do.

With CFS, the path is rarely straight forward. But even in the middle of chaos, things may go forward. You can measure it and, at the same time, comprehend the shortcomings by documenting.

You are compiling a chronology of your health with each entry. This timeline eventually turns into a reflection tool and a source of hope; no matter how small the steps are, progress will be evident throughout the pages.

One patient shared with me her "record of minor victories," a compilation of instances in which she experienced a glimmer of her previous energy. Her writings of these occasions served as talismans to keep her from giving up.

Your journey, once chronicled, can remind you of how far you've gone, which can be comforting and inspire you to keep going when things become tough.

In the intricate dance of CFS management, dialogue with your medical team is essential. The choreography is provided by your recorded insights.

Your notes can facilitate more in-depth discussions with your physicians and therapists, resulting in more individualised treatment. We can precisely adjust your treatment plan with the assistance of the details you supply.

Patients who bring their diaries to consultations frequently feel accomplished after having an informed and fruitful discussion regarding their health.

Just showing your documented experiences could make all the difference in your next appointment. This gives you and your healthcare practitioner the ability to make knowledgeable decisions.

Writing can be a cathartic process that releases emotional baggage from the soul.

Your journal's pages can turn into a safe haven for your ideas and emotions, a place where you can express yourself without fear of rejection or shame.

Many people have found comfort in writing in their journals, expressing the sense of release they get from putting their hearts on paper.

Think of your notebook as a friend that will listen to you without interjecting, giving you the room you need to heal both physically and emotionally.

Knowledge is your ally, and you become its carrier by documenting it. You are equipped to speak up for your own health and wellbeing if you keep up a well-kept notebook.

Knowing the features of your illness gives you a voice. You can use this voice to ask for accommodations, communicate your requirements to family and friends, or join the growing number of people who are advocating for more public awareness of CFS.

I've seen patients talk more clearly and stand taller more often because of their personal experiences.

Enformed by your diary, your self-advocacy can lead to better understanding and care, whether at a doctor's office or social event.

As we move from point to point, the general reality emerges: recording your experience with CFS is an act of self-care, a management technique, and a basis for empowerment. It is not just a record-keeping exercise.

The pen in your hand is a very powerful instrument. With it, you may map out the features of your illness, write a storey about your perseverance, and negotiate the difficulties associated with chronic fatigue syndrome. Once shrouded in mystery, your journey might become clear page by page, telling a brave, perceptive, and hopeful tale. Accept this practise because it is a road map to mastery, not just a journal.

The Road to Recovery: Stories of Hope

Overcoming Challenges

The Resilient Path Forward

—-

I have seen people go through my doors and experience deep victories and silent battles during the calm mornings at my practise, when the sun shines softly over the dew-kissed trees. Chronic fatigue syndrome, or CFS, is more than just a disease; it's a relentless wave that challenges one's ability to persevere. Allow me to tell you a storey about human resiliency and triumph in addition to suffering.

Our hero is Sarah, a graphic designer whose vibrant talent once influenced her life. Up until CFS threw a shadow over her canvas, she was the picture of health. The main obstacle Sarah had to overcome was extreme exhaustion—the kind that confines a person to bed and makes days seem like a haze of exhaustion.

The treatment for Sarah's CFS was multimodal, as any multimodal condition should be given to cover all facets of a person's life. We plotted a route that involved careful meal preparation, incorporating nutrients that reduce inflammation and increase vitality. We talked about the psychological effects of CFS in counselling, where Sarah could express her feelings, and we looked at body- and mind-inclusive self-care practises.

Our plan changed over time, adapting to Sarah's demands in the same way that a willow bends with the wind. Though they took time to manifest, the effects were real. Sarah started to retrieve the hours she had lost due to CFS, connecting them as though they were pearls of hope on a healing necklace. She claimed feeling less tired as well as having more control over her life.

Looking back on Sarah's experience, it's clear that every person's journey toward treating CFS is different. The lessons learned here should not be interpreted as prescriptions, but rather as markers indicating areas for development and stressing the value of an individualised strategy.

Visual tools, such a weekly diet plan or a graph showing Sarah's energy levels, could help to show the methodical and progressive nature of her recovery strategy.

Sarah's narrative represents a one strand in the larger picture of CFS care. By emphasising the value of a holistic approach—one that treats the syndrome's emotional and psychological components in addition to its physical manifestation—it ties into the book's overall storey.

So as you flip the page, my dear reader, allow me to leave you with this thought to ponder: What tiny action can you take today that can result in a better tomorrow?

Recall that managing chronic fatigue syndrome is a marathon that calls for perseverance, fortitude, and a customised plan. Let's be motivated to forge our way to wellness with hope and determination as we work through 'The Chronic Fatigue Syndrome Mastery Bible: Your Blueprint for Complete Chronic Fatigue Syndrome Management', taking inspiration from stories like Sarah's.

Adapting and Thriving

Imagine living in a world where waking up each morning is a daunting task and the act itself signals the start of a day filled with uncertainty. This is the scene that many people who suffer from Chronic Fatigue Syndrome (CFS) play out their everyday lives against. Nevertheless, there are those in this scene of hardship who have not only adapted but even thrived.

Let me introduce you to Maya, a lively graphic designer whose life was completely turned upside down when CFS struck. Maya, who was once a ball of energy, was now faced with an unseen enemy that was eating away at her energy and making her feel alienated from her own existence. Her storey embodies the fundamental difficulty experienced by people with CFS: finding a way to restore a feeling of purpose and normalcy in the face of constant exhaustion.

Maya's approach consisted on small changes and unwavering resolve rather than big showy gestures. Together with my team, we designed a plan that combined dietary planning, lifestyle adjustments, and mental toughness. We set out on a holistic journey to realign Maya's life together.

The strategy was diverse since, similar to CFS, the remedies needed to be flexible and dynamic. We started a symphony of changes, including mindful techniques to ground her in the present, nutrient-rich food to restore her depleted resources, and moderate yoga to build physical resilience. The outcome was a slow reawakening rather than an abrupt transformation.

Weeks turned into months, and Maya's life started to resurface like the first glimmer of dawn after a long night. She reported a forty percent reduction in daily exhaustion and a thirty percent improvement in energy levels. The data was positive. It served as evidence of the effectiveness of a comprehensive strategy.

However, we must not eliminate reflection from our analysis. Innumerable Mayas are adrift in the turbulent waters of CFS for every Maya. Even though they work, our tactics are not a cure-all. Every journey is different, and achieving wellness requires patience and tenacity.

Visual aids, like Maya's record of her energy and exhaustion, functioned as a guide and a mirror. We could make necessary adjustments to our techniques in real time, making sure that every step forward was based on her lived experience, by monitoring her progress.

Maya's storey is only one part of the greater storey of CFS. It emphasises the main idea of this book, which is that managing CFS is a difficult but manageable task that calls for a well-balanced combination of medical knowledge and guts.

Are you able to relate to Maya's storey? Is it possible for you to picture a similar course of growth and adaptation in your own life?

A paradigm change is required to adjust to CFS; one must reimagine their life within the constraints of a new reality. It necessitates learning to appreciate the body's limits, pacing technique, and rhythm. It's about developing an encouraging and compassionate inner dialogue and discovering happiness in the little things.

Redefining what success looks like is the key to thriving with CFS, though. It's about enjoying the peace of a calm afternoon, something that the busyness of a previous life could never have allowed, or it's about honouring the capacity to work on significant projects, even if it's only for a few hours each day.

Ultimately, mastering Chronic Fatigue Syndrome is more than just treating its symptoms; it's about rewriting the storey of your life so that you are the strong, resilient lead who skillfully rides out its ups and downs.

I'd want to leave you with this idea: What tiny action can you do today to plant the seeds of your own tale of thriving and adapting?

Remember that the journey with CFS is both incredibly personal and shared by all as we wrap up this subchapter. Many others have gone before you, and by leaning on their wisdom and your own inner fortitude, you too may steer clear of CFS's constraints and toward the limitless possibilities of the human spirit.

Holistic Success Stories

Imagine, if you will, a world where the exhausted find strength, the weary find respite, and the bright colours of life are revealed when the fog of exhaustion lifts. In my years of practise, I have guided a great number of people—people who had previously been trapped by the unrelenting clutches of chronic fatigue syndrome—through this life-changing experience (CFS). This subsection, cherished peruser, honours their triumphs and bears witness to the potency of all-encompassing recovery.

Allow me to present Maya to you. Maya used to be an enthusiastic hiker, but her life took an unexpected turn when CFS cast a pall over her days with unwavering fatigue. Her previously sharp and concentrated intellect clouded over. She was not at all happy about the prospect of a mountain trail.

Maya's main struggle was complex, combining social seclusion, emotional upheaval, and physical weakness. Her condition had been diagnosed by the conventional medical method, but there was no apparent cure. This marked the start of our holistic journey.

We set out on a journey that combined mindfulness, diet, and modest physical reconditioning. My team and I, consisting of a psychologist, physical therapist, and dietitian, created a customised lifestyle plan for Maya. Her erratic diet was replaced with nutrient-dense meals, and she started doing breathing exercises and meditation every day. Her physical therapist introduced her to a progressive training regimen that honoured the limitations of her body.

The outcome? Though they took time to materialise, Maya's energy started to bloom once more as the weeks passed into months. Her sleep deepened, her endurance increased, and the long-overdue cerebral fog started to lift. One step at a time, she was taking back her life.

When one considers Maya's journey, it becomes evident that she achieved success in more ways than one. She had greater emotional resilience. She made new connections on a social level and finally discovered her way back to the trails she cherished. Though the evidence was strong—better sleep, more activity, and a marked decline in her tiredness score—her radiant smile and the glimmer in her eyes revealed the real extent of her achievement.

Her symptom diaries and progress charts, among other visual tools, provided concrete benchmarks for her progress. They served as evidence of her commitment and the effectiveness of a wholistic strategy.

Maya's tale is only one strand in an intricate web of lives that have been changed. Despite the differences in each storey, they all speak to the same truth: the importance of treating the whole person rather than just the symptoms. The greater storey of holistic health, which weaves like a golden thread throughout this book, is connected to us through these stories.

What if the element missing from your CFS treatment puzzle was something you could also find?

Think about Akash, a talented musician whose symphonies were drowned out by the noise of CFS. Along with his psychological conflicts, the demands of the music industry—to compose, perform, and be present in its unrelenting rhythm—also played a major role in his life.

In addition to dietary changes and physical therapy, Akash's treatment plan included sound therapy and stress reduction. We looked at how music may be used therapeutically, transforming his own love into a tool for healing. Reduced anxiety, enhanced cognitive function, and a gradual return to composition were the remarkable outcomes.

As you consider these tales, keep in mind that there are many ways to achieve wellbeing rather than just one, which is the basis of holistic health care. Every journey is a patchwork of setbacks, victories, and learnings.

However, may I ask you how your mosaic appears? Have you figured out the parts that make up your wellness?

Finally, remember that although these triumphant tales serve as motivation, the path to effectively treating CFS is seldom straight-forward. It's a journey of learning and unlearning, of peaks and valleys. I want you to think about your personal storey as we turn the page to the next chapter. Which tactics will you use, and which accomplishments will you acknowledge?

Recall that achieving health is a marathon, not a sprint, and that the holistic approach will be your constant comrade, helping you cross the finish line with the medals of vitality and wellbeing.

Medical Breakthroughs

Envision a society in which the arduous entanglement of Chronic Fatigue Syndrome (CFS) is lifted from the lives of those it affects. As a ray of hope in this sometimes misunderstood field, I, Dr. Ankita Kashyap, have personally seen the life-changing potential of medical advancements in the treatment of CFS.

Allow me to take you to a small clinic tucked away in the middle of a busy metropolis, where holistic therapy methods coexist with conventional medicine to provide a special haven for people suffering with CFS. One face sticks out among the multitude of others looking for assistance: Sarah, a 34-year-old graphic designer whose life was once colourful and active but was now obscured by a lingering cloud of exhaustion.

Many people can relate to Sarah's storey because she was previously active and is now struggling with the debilitating effects of CFS. The difficulty? to return Sarah to her life prior to CFS's shadow being cast over her.

Our strategy was diverse, which is indicative of the integrated healthcare model that forms the basis of our business. We examined Sarah's food, lifestyle, and mental health using a variety of approaches, from cutting-edge self-help methods to evidence-based medical interventions. These weren't only therapies; they were steps toward getting back control over her health.

The outcome? An insight. Sarah's energy started to come back, her soul revived. The genuine picture of success was created by the resurgence of her creative spark, her ability to stay up late, and her renewed hope; numbers alone are unable to adequately convey such a metamorphosis.

When one considers Sarah's experience, it becomes evident that managing CFS is not a simple process. Trial and error, tenacity, and most importantly, an unwavering spirit of discovery are the paving stones of this journey. Although some may contest the anecdotal character of these case studies, they represent indisputable evidence of the possibility for advancement and the effectiveness of individualised treatment.

Visual aids, like Sarah's symptom log, helped to translate her subjective experience into a real narrative by illustrating the significant changes over time. These resources not only improved her comprehension but also gave her the confidence to take an active role in her recovery.

Sarah's narrative is a single strand within the broader fabric of CFS care. It's a storey that resonates with the main concepts of this book: the unwavering belief that every instance can lead to new opportunities for wellness and vitality, and the unwavering goal of control over CFS.

Now, please take a time to relax, reader. Is it possible for you to envision a life in which CFS is only a memory?

We are now moving from the particular to the general in our discussion. Modern medicine is producing ground breaking discoveries at a rate never seen before, and these discoveries have the power to completely change the face of CFS. The future is full of possibilities, ranging from brand-new gene therapy uses to cutting-edge pharmaceutical therapies.

But what does this mean for you?

It represents a time when treating CFS will involve more than just symptom management. It signals a time when the goal of treatment is to help patients thrive rather than just get by.

You will learn about the many ways that holistic healing methods and scientific discoveries blend together to create a symphony of healing possibilities as we travel through this trip together. Every chapter you read and every tale you take in will provide you with the skills you need to create your own management roadmap for CFS.

Let's pause to consider this: what if the pages you are holding actually contain the secret to reviving your life?

In summary, the tales of medical advances in the treatment of chronic fatigue syndrome are more than just clinical case studies; they represent a ray of hope. They are the sparks that light the way to a life regained by igniting the flame of possibilities. As we wrap up this chapter, let's spread the awareness that every discovery we make brings us one step closer to understanding the mystery of chronic fatigue syndrome.

Thus, I extend an optimistic heartfelt invitation for you to flip the page. Together, let's keep deciphering the riddles behind CFS and pave the way for healing and vigour that previously appeared unachievable.

Learning From Setbacks

Setbacks are not just roadblocks in the maze-like management of Chronic Fatigue Syndrome (CFS); rather, they are the unseen markers pointing the way toward understanding and resilience. Think back to a case that has stayed with me, one that demonstrates the enduring strength of human resilience and the transforming potential of complementary medicine.

Set the Scene

For many, the sun-dappled consulting room with its jasmine aroma and calming music hum served as a haven. People struggling with the mysterious shadow of CFS found comfort and answers here.

Introduce the Main Players

Here comes Sarah, a once-bright graphic designer whose life was a creative canvas that has been dimmed by the never-ending mist of exhaustion. She was once a ray of unending energy, but the unforgiving winds of CFS left her adrift in the sea of fatigue.

Present the Challenge or Problem

Sarah faced many difficulties on her path. Her energy fluctuated so much that each day was like a gamble. Even though she adhered to the carefully designed treatment plan, she suffered a depressing setback: months of improvement were reversed by a relapse brought on by an acute viral illness.

Detail the Approach or Solution

Following this depressing development, we assembled our team, which included professionals with backgrounds in psychology, nutrition, and alternative medicine. A customised strategy was developed, considering Sarah's particular situation. In order to support her physical and mental equilibrium, we added moderate yoga and immune-boosting foods to her diet. We used cognitive-behavioral strategies to protect her from the psychological effects of her illness.

Showcase the Results

The results of this multifaceted strategy started to show over time. Sarah's reserves of energy were no longer permanently depleted. Her recovery represented an ascension to a new level of wellbeing rather than just a return to baseline.

Analyze and Reflect

However, it would be incorrect to say there were no barriers in the way. Every stride forward was a risky dance, but it was this same dance that imparted the most important lessons to us. Sarah's experience demonstrates that in the world of CFS, obstacles are not final; rather, they are turning points in a person's life where holistic intervention can change course.

Visual Aids (if applicable)

Sarah's journey may have been represented graphically as a graph with peaks and valleys, but overall it was a trend of inspiration, a visual hymn to the resilience of the human spirit.

Connect to the Larger Narrative or Concept

Sarah's storey is a microcosm of the larger storey that captures the spirit of CFS care. It is a storey spun from strands of hardship, resiliency, and victory. It speaks to the essence of our purpose, which is to use holistic wisdom as an anchor and medical science as a compass to navigate the choppy waters of CFS.

Transition Thought or Question

In tackling the mystery of CFS, what does Sarah's experience teach us about the interaction of the body, mind, and spirit?

Living with Chronic Fatigue Syndrome is like painting on a canvas that is always shifting and occasionally smeared by unintentional brushstrokes. But it's in these smudges that we reveal our genuine selves, our ability to change, and our ability to turn failures into opportunities for success.

Variety is essential to participation, so as we navigate the CFS environment, let's make the most of the wide range of resources at our disposal. Have you thought about how meditation affects your journey, the quiet symphony that soothes the turbulent waves of exhaustion?

Adjectives and adverbs are only the garnish for our story's filling dinner; the real food is found in the strong nouns and verbs, the concrete components of our all-encompassing strategy.

One sentence can serve as a sentinel and a truth-keeper: Reversals are not a sign of failure but rather of progress and in-depth learning.

That which is truly wise is simple. The path forward in managing CFS is not determined by the intricacy of our strategy, but rather by the clarity of our intentions.

Our conversational pace reflects the ebb and flow of energy in a CFS patient, which is a tapestry of highs and lows stitched with compassion and understanding.

As Sarah once said, "In this journey, I've not only learned to manage my energy but to appreciate it, to honour it, and to invest it in what actually counts," quotations provide life to our storey.

If there is one lesson to be learned from Sarah's tale, it is this: mastering chronic fatigue syndrome is a constant journey rather than a destination, one that is characterised by learning from setbacks, adapting techniques, and, most importantly, an unwavering commitment to wellbeing.

Now, as you turn the page, dear reader, consider this: What obstacles have you faced, and how have they influenced your journey to become an expert in CFS?

The Importance of Perseverance

Perseverance is an essential ally in the complex process of managing Chronic Fatigue Syndrome (CFS), not just a virtue. Let's use Maya's tale to help brighten the route as we make our way through the thick fog of CFS. She is more than just a case study; she is evidence of the human spirit's tenacity.

Set the Scene:

In a fast-paced metropolis, where everything happens at the speed of light, there once was Maya, a dynamic professional with goals as lofty as the surrounding skyscrapers. The city, a flurry of activity, is unaffected by her abrupt conflict with CFS, an unseen foe.

Introduce the Main Players:

The primary characters in this storey are Maya, who is adjusting to her new life; her network of friends, family, and coworkers; and my team, which is made up of medical experts committed to holistic health.

Present the Challenge or Problem:

Maya faced several challenges, including the psychological effects of an unpredictable illness, the physical debilitation brought on by CFS, and the social isolation resulting from others' lack of understanding.

Detail the Approach or Solution:

Our plan took a comprehensive approach, putting equal emphasis on promoting Maya's mental and emotional health as well as symptom treatment. We customised a programme of nutritional adjustments, holistic self-care techniques, and counselling.

Showcase the Results:

Months passed, and Maya's perseverance paid off. She reported feeling more in control of her life, having more energy, and having more mental clarity. CFS was still there in her storey, but it was no longer the pen.

Analyze and Reflect:

Even though Maya's development was encouraging, it's important to recognise that every person's experience with CFS is different. Not every tactic is effective in every situation, and persistence does not ensure a straight line to progress.

Visual Aids (if applicable):

Envision a graph that includes plateaus in addition to peaks and troughs—points where Maya's advancement remained constant, demonstrating to us that steadiness is also growth.

Connect to the Larger Narrative or Concept:

Maya's narrative is just one small part of the CFS management puzzle. It emphasises a universal truth: flexibility and tenacity go hand in hand in perseverance.

Transition Thought or Question:

Think about your path while you analyse Maya's trip. How does tenacity manifest itself in your life with CFS?

—-

Chronic fatigue syndrome, or CFS, is a multifaceted and sometimes misdiagnosed illness that is typified by a wide range of symptoms that can severely disrupt daily activities in addition to persistent fatigue. In these pages, we examine the ways in which tenacity—that unshakable resolve—is an essential component of the CFS management puzzle. Isn't it amazing how the human soul perseveres when the physical body fails?

Think about Maya's experience, a case that will always be remembered in the history of my work. Her journey from the depths of hopelessness to taking back her storey is instructive as well as inspirational. Join me as we explore how tenacity combined with complementary medicine might be a ray of hope for people stumbling through the murky seas of CFS.

It was a regular Monday morning when Maya's storey started. Her life was organised to a rhythm that was the cacophony of the city, her symphony. However, the music faded as CFS set in and was replaced with the droning thud of tiredness. Her life, once a colourful fresco, now looked like a canvas wiped clean by the never-ending downpour of exhaustion.

Maya, a representation of tenacity, stood in the middle. Her friends were the sideline cheerleaders; her family was a comforting sanctuary; and her coworkers were the unaware onlookers. And then there was us, a group of medical professionals, ready to assist her in taking back her life.

Relieving the physical symptoms—which included constant fatigue, discomfort, and mental fog—was not the only problem. Additionally, it was intended to heal the invisible wounds of CFS, which frequently include frustration, worry, and despair.

It wasn't a one-size-fits-all strategy. Adapting our strategy to Maya's requirements, we included nutrient-dense meal planning to help her fight off exhaustion. We incorporated self-care practises while fostering the body-mind connection. We tackled therapy head-on, removing the psychological burden that CFS frequently carries.

The outcome? They took some time to appear. It's a marathon, not a sprint, to persevere. However, Maya started to notice a change as the weeks stretched into months. Her energy levels, which were previously dependent on CFS, occasionally defied them. She started to see flashes of the clarity she had taken for granted as her mental fog started to clear.

But it's crucial to consider the characteristics of this creature we refer to as CFS. Not all progress is linear. A part of the trip are setbacks. But real development is gained when persistence is steady and one refuses to let the condition define them.

Consider Maya's progress chart, if you will. It's not just a straight line upward. The network of peaks, troughs, and plateaus is intricate. However, every dot on that graph denotes a day she made the decision to press on—a choice that by itself is symbolic of success.

Maya's storey is just one colour on the spectrum of experiences related to CFS. It shows us that perseverance is more than just overcoming obstacles; it's also about changing and coming up with fresh strategies for overcoming life's obstacles. It serves as a reminder that sometimes standing your ground is just as admirable as moving forward.

As we get to the end of Maya's journey, I want you to consider the struggles you have had with CFS. What does persistence mean to you? Is it a resolute march forward or a soft acceptance of where you are right now combined with the will to keep trying and keeping hoping?

We set out on a journey toward not just management but also mastery with the help of this book, "The Chronic Fatigue Syndrome Mastery Bible: Your Blueprint for Complete Chronic Fatigue Syndrome Management." Because tolerating, adapting, and thriving are just as important as overcoming in the art of living with CFS.

Messages of Encouragement

I've seen adventures that leave me in amazement, all within the peaceful sanctuary of my practise, where the soft hum of life whispers tales of resilience. I met Maya there, among the lush vegetation that seems to cradle life itself. Maya was a lively person whose life was suddenly interrupted by the deafening quiet caused by Chronic Fatigue Syndrome (CFS). Like many others, her storey is marked by the anguish of days lost, but it also serves as a monument to the human spirit's tenacity.

That was an average Thursday, the kind when everything goes around in a predictable circle and nobody pays any attention to the mayhem that is going to take place in one person's life. Her days as a graphic designer and a mother of two were a colourful collage of deadlines, colours, and laughter—that is, until CFS cast its shadow and made her life an endless search for energy.

The task at hand was both evident and intimidating. Maya's CFS showed up as constant exhaustion, fogginess in her head, and discomfort that didn't go away with rest. Her illness, which was frequently misinterpreted, made her feel alone in a world that was passing by too quickly.

We took a comprehensive approach to Maya's situation in our healing sanctuary. Our team, which included psychiatrists and dietitians, created a customised treatment plan for her. We stitched together a diet of nutrient-dense meals, counselling sessions, and lifestyle changes to help her express her frustrations and worries.

Even though they weren't instantaneous, the outcomes were a patchwork of tiny wins. Maya's energy continued to nudge upward, her discomfort started to become less of a companion, and the fog in her head started to clear, exposing the bright mind underneath. Week by week, Maya retrieved pieces of her old self, assembling them into a mosaic of optimism.

Thinking back on Maya's journey makes me realise how carefully patience and action must tango together. Although there isn't a miracle treatment for CFS, there is a way to manage the condition better with a customised approach.

For a brief minute, consider the courage required to confront every day with the knowledge that your own body appears to be against you. Imagine now having the bravery to keep on in spite of everything. This is the core of every word of inspiration I want to share.

Do you not think, reader, that this kind of resiliency is simply amazing?

As I write this, I realise very clearly that CFS is a large canvas on which every person has painted a unique portrait of struggle and victory. There is a continuum, and no two experiences are exactly the same. Nonetheless, what unites us is the essence of our common human experience.

I cordially encourage you to explore more into the core of this book in the spirit of connectivity. The techniques, perceptions, and collective knowledge are all only means of assisting you in navigating your individual CFS journey.

Think about this: What modest action can you take now that you will be grateful for later?

Moving from Maya's tale to the global fight against CFS, let's keep in mind that every setback is an opportunity for growth and every triumph is a result of overcoming adversity. This subsection merely serves as an introduction to the symphony of tactics and narratives that await you within these pages.

Now that we have been strengthened by Maya's tale and our minds are full of ideas on how we might become experts at managing our Chronic Fatigue Syndrome, let's flip the page.

We travel this route together, one that is filled with healing, optimism, and the unwavering quest of wellbeing.

Conclusion: Embracing a New Normal

Summarizing Key Strategies

As dawn rises on a new day, so too does the prospect of controlling Chronic Fatigue Syndrome (CFS) manifest itself with appropriate tactics. Greetings, readers. My name is Dr. Ankita Kashyap, and what you will find in these pages is the essence of my approach—a holistic symphony that masterfully blends the best notes of wellness coaching and medical knowledge.

Let's stop at the threshold and compile our road map of essential tactics before navigating the maze of CFS management. The list that follows is not just a how-to manual; rather, it is a lighthouse that points you in the direction of better health and energy.

1. Lifestyle Modifications
2. Nutritional Optimization
3. Psychological Empowerment
4. Self-Care Rituals
5. Coping Mechanisms

The Rhythm of Routine

Your life's pace is determined by your daily schedule. Rearranging your daily routine can help you feel more in control, be more productive, and preserve energy when CFS is acting up.

Evidence and Testimonials

Patients like Sarah, who at one point felt lost in the ocean of exhaustion, learned that making small adjustments—making sleep a priority, timing activities, and including light exercise—can provide stability in one's life during a difficult time.

Practical Applications

How would you put these changes into practise? Think about the benefits of maintaining a healing sleep routine and arranging your workload so that it fits your energy levels.

The Alchemy of Eating

Food is the alchemist's stone that can change your health, it's more than just nourishment. Every meal becomes an opportunity to nourish and heal for someone with CFS.

Evidence and Testimonials

Studies highlight the connection between gut health and overall wellness, and many like Raj have recovered their energy by consuming anti-inflammatory foods and following customised diet regimens.

Practical Applications

Think of your plate as a brilliant colour palette, with each bite serving as a brushstroke that adds to your masterpiece of health. Accept whole foods, make the most of staying hydrated, and allow your body to absorb the nutrients.

Conversations with the Self

Your storey about your health has an impact on how you deal with CFS. You have the power to change the course of your life by utilising psychological strategies.

Evidence and Testimonials

For many, the way has been lighted by mindfulness and cognitive-behavioral therapy (CBT). Consider James, whose struggle with CFS improved after he adopted these techniques that promoted optimism and resilience.

Practical Applications

Whether you use journaling, meditation, or therapy, invite these conversations into your life. Talk to yourself in a positive and uplifting way since you have unlimited influence over your thoughts.

Crafting Moments of Serenity

Self-care serves as your little haven where you can escape the chaos of CFS. It's the skill of creating experiences that uplift and revitalise the soul.

Evidence and Testimonials

Emma's storey of experiencing the peace of warm baths and the comfort of yoga highlights the transforming potential of self-care practises.

Practical Applications

Create your haven using techniques that you find meaningful, such as aromatherapy, yoga, or deep breathing. Allow every routine to serve as a thread in the overall design of your wellbeing.

The Compass of Resilience

Coping strategies serve as your compass on the uncertain journey towards resilience in the face of CFS.

Evidence and Testimonials

Many people have found strength in community and adaptability, as seen by individuals like Anand, for whom support groups and adaptable tactics have been lifesavers.

Practical Applications

Become a part of support systems, make reasonable goals, and acknowledge little accomplishments as ways to find your compass. Every advance is a victory.

The symphony of managing Chronic Fatigue Syndrome truly resonates when all the strategies work together, even though each one sings its own unique note. I am your guide, and I am here to lead this holistic health opera with you at the helm of the orchestra.

Have you sensed the need to change your way of life, to experience the bliss of perfect nourishment, to strengthen your intellect, to engage in self-care, and to learn how to handle difficult situations with grace? If so, let these pages serve as your guide and inspiration.

Go deeper, my dear reader, for this book contains friendship as well as tactics for achieving mastery. Together, with hopes bursting from our hearts and spirits unbroken by weariness, let's set off on this voyage.

Maintaining Hope and Positivity

Maintaining optimism and hope is not only a comforting balm but also a crucial compass for navigating the murky seas of Chronic Fatigue Syndrome (CFS), a labyrinth where every corridor appears to resound with fatigue. Turn the pages of this chapter and join us as we set out to explore the potential of a positive outlook on the long-term care of CFS.

For a brief instant, picture a world in which the exhaustion that seeps into your bones is only a passing shadow. That is appealing, isn't it? However, this is a far-off goal for many people, clouded by the reality of CFS. Here, the obvious main obstacle is how to cultivate hope in the face of energy's apparent scarcity.

If you give up on this pursuit of happiness, the results will be severe. A depressive spiral can make symptoms worse, impair judgement, and close doors that could otherwise result in improved health. However, we are not helpless in this conflict. As a holistic health and wellness coach, I have seen firsthand the transformation that positivity can bring about.

What then is the remedy? It is found in using our own mental faculties. Thoughts have a significant impact on our physical health; this relationship is often overlooked but is unquestionably potent.

Daily affirmations are the first easy but important step in putting this method into practise. As the globe awakens every morning, declare your dedication to optimism. "Today, I choose action over inaction, optimism over despair." Allow these words to serve as the cornerstone of your day.

Add to your routine by keeping a thankfulness diary as well. Every night, as the sky becomes covered in stars, list three things for which you are thankful. This exercise centres you in the here and now and shifts your attention from your problems to your benefits.

There is more than just anecdotal evidence to support the effectiveness of positive thinking; research has demonstrated that it can enhance physical health. Patients who keep a positive outlook frequently report feeling more in control of their situation and experiencing fewer symptoms.

However, it would be imprudent to assert that this is the only path through CFS. Other remedies include mindfulness meditation, which strengthens the bond between the mind and body, and cognitive-behavioral therapy (CBT), which restructures harmful thought patterns. On this journey towards well-being, both are deserving allies.

I would like to know whether you have ever observed how one optimistic idea in the morning may change the entire trajectory of your day?

Imagine the brilliant colours of a dawn, a constant reminder that every day is a blank canvas waiting for your optimistic brushstrokes. This vision is meant to instil in your mind the possibilities that each new day brings, not just to paint a lovely picture.

You may be asking yourself by now what concrete steps I can take to keep this positive attitude. These are a handful:

- Be in a group of people who are encouraging to you. Your personal hope can be amplified by the resonance of common experiences.

- Establish tiny but attainable goals. Every success serves as a lighthouse for advancement.

- Look for joy in the ordinary. The things that kindle hope are a favourite song, a fit of giggles, and the peace of nature.

Remember that simplicity is your ally in the fight to hold onto optimism. While intricate plans may seem overwhelming, small, regular acts of kindness create strongholds of optimism.

Living with CFS may have an erratic rhythm, but you don't have to let it dictate how you react to it. Discover your balance and move to the pulse of optimism by following the rhythm of these exercises.

Helen Keller, a shining example of overcoming hardship, once said, "Optimism is the faith that brings success. Without confidence and hope, nothing is possible." Allow her words to reverberate within your heart while you navigate CFS management.

In summary, staying upbeat and hopeful is not just a nice idea—it is an essential tactic in controlling chronic fatigue syndrome. Let the spirit of positivity lead the way as you turn the pages of this comprehensive CFS management roadmap, shedding light on the way ahead with every step you take. Accept this trip as a group experience rather than a solo one, where hope is the light that endures through the darkest of circumstances.

The Role of Acceptance

Sarah was sitting in a quiet room, her silhouette a symbol of strength against the gentle glow of dawn. Her experience with Chronic Fatigue Syndrome (CFS) was characterised by a multitude of difficulties, a trip across turbulent waters of doubt and hopelessness. However, her storey also reveals a profound truth about the power of acceptance, which is like a beacon pointing a ship toward land.

The unwavering hold of CFS upset Sarah's life's rhythm; she was once an unstoppable marathon runner. Her new enemy was the sneaky start of chronic fatigue that no amount of sleep could defeat. She carried an unseen burden, her life evaporating from her fingertips like sand grains.

The main struggle Sarah faced was coming to terms with this unexpected, new chapter in her life's narrative rather than just dealing with the physical symptoms that CFS brought on. Could the dissonant sounds of her illness reconcile her spirit?

Sarah sought the advice of our integrated wellness experts to help her through this journey. We set out on a painstakingly customised path together, fusing medical expertise with the entire tapestry of mind-body-soul healing. Our strategy was to look for harmony and balance inside the storm rather than a cure-all.

Customized lifestyle adjustments were her daily mantras, and a harmonic balance of nutritional meals catered to her body's requirements. Her safe havens, where she could untangle the strands of her feelings, were counselling sessions. Through practising self-compassion and mindfulness, Sarah gradually learned to accept the fluctuations in her energy levels and realised that her value was not dependent on how productive she was.

Our joint symphony with Sarah produced tremendous outcomes. Her experiences started to take on different hues, even while CFS continued to be a part of her life. Her acceptance opened the door for empowerment and a renewed sense of control rather than defeat. Sarah continued to find moments of calm and moments of joy that had seemed to have vanished into the abyss with every day that went by.

When one considers Sarah's journey, it becomes clear that accepting reality is an active process rather than a passive surrender. It is the beginning of the change process. Without acceptance, we are always at odds with the unalterable, diverting our energies from recovery and development.

Sarah's energy diary, a graphical depiction of her highs and lows, was one of the visual tools that demonstrated her development. These weren't just any charts; they were ink-etched representations of her acceptance and resiliency.

For anyone attempting to navigate the murky seas of CFS, Sarah's storey serves as a beacon. It ties in with our book's overall storey by highlighting how crucial acceptance is to treating long-term illnesses. It serves as the base for all other tactics and the fertile ground where wellness seeds grow.

So how do we develop this essential component of acceptance in our own lives? It all begins with a small but significant adjustment in viewpoint—a readiness to recognise our experiences and pay attention to our bodies.

As we conclude this storey of resiliency, let us consider the following inquiry, which is both an invitation and a challenge: What facets of our own lives—whether or not they are impacted by CFS—are we resisting, and how might acceptance hold the key to revealing a more profound sense of purpose and serenity?

When it comes to Chronic Fatigue Syndrome, acceptance is a journey rather than a goal. It is a delicate waltz between our aspirations and our circumstances, and when it is accepted, it can result in a life lived with elegance and intention.

Thus, let us keep the memory of Sarah's bravery with us as we close this chapter of her life. Since acceptance is the first step toward conquering chronic fatigue syndrome, let's make room in our own lives for it. We are never really lost when we use acceptance as our compass since it points us in the direction of our inner strength and tranquilly.

Finally, as you peruse the pages of "The Chronic Fatigue Syndrome Mastery Bible," keep in mind that every tactic and piece of guidance is but one strand in the greater fabric of your recovery process. The cornerstone, the base upon which you can construct a life that is informed and enhanced by your condition rather than defined by it, is acceptance. Accept this path, as it is special to you and has the possibility of significant change.

Continuing Education and Advocacy

Chronic fatigue syndrome, or CFS, is a disease that is often poorly understood in the maze of chronic conditions. As a wellness coach and medical practitioner, I have witnessed the ignorance and mishandling of this illness. Patients come to me with tales of years lost to extreme exhaustion that keeps them confined to their beds, of treatments that fall short of expectations, and of disbelief from people they trusted. These tragedies are not isolated incidents; rather, they serve as an urgent cry for greater understanding and a stronger network of support.

Take a moment to reflect on the widespread effects of CFS, a disorder that affects millions of people worldwide and shows little regard for boundaries. It is a time-thief, taking away one's most fruitful years, but many people in the medical field and society at general still don't understand it. What if they continue to be ignorant? The result is disastrous: people keep suffering in silence, cures are still elusive, and the cycle of misinformation keeps going.

Two strategies are needed to solve the problem: constant advocacy and education. Together, they provide as the cornerstone of transformation for people affected by CFS. Patients, healthcare professionals, and the general public are empowered by education, and research and policy reforms are pushed for by advocacy, which increases the collective voice. Gaining more knowledge is not the only goal; applying that knowledge to accomplish more is.

The first step in putting this plan into practise is distributing current, reliable information regarding CFS. Enlightening the general public and healthcare professionals about the intricacies of this disease can be accomplished through workshops, seminars, and online courses. These learning resources need to be interesting, accurate, and easily available. In my capacity as your reliable advisor, I promise to provide materials that capture this philosophy and offer perspectives from the nexus of holistic health care and medical science.

There is ample proof of the effectiveness of campaigning and education. Think about the advancements achieved in other chronic disorders that were formerly stigmatised and mysterious. When people banded together, information proliferated, medical advances were made, and lives were recovered. For CFS, we anticipate a similar trajectory as knowledge and awareness increase.

Of course, advocacy is just as important as education; neither is a cure-all. advocacy that calls for financing for the creation of thorough treatment regimens, patient support services, and research. It cries out for action and does not mutter; rather, it roars.

So why not form a coalition of medical professionals, patients, and supporters to advocate for reform? We can effectively communicate the necessity for research money and the inclusion of CFS in medical curriculum by speaking with one voice. Together, we can create petitions, visit with lawmakers, and use social media to further our cause.

However, one can ponder if there are other options. Individual efforts, like personal blogs and neighbourhood support groups, undoubtedly have a significant impact. They provide comfort and support, but they also need to work in tandem with larger initiatives to change the perception of CFS.

Imagine a society in which CFS is no longer a diagnosis to be whispered about, but rather a challenge to be tackled with all of our knowledge and compassion. a setting in which patients receive nods of understanding rather than confused shrugs. Through activism and education, we hope to bring about this kind of world.

We have to work tirelessly to accomplish this. Investment is necessary, including of time, money, and passion. Ready to take part in this movement? To take a stand with people who are unable to stand by themselves?

And so, as we proceed, the management blueprint for CFS becomes a live document that changes with every new finding and every anecdote that is shared, rather than merely a list of rules. It's a journey that goes beyond the self and touches the core of our humanity, community, and society.

Ultimately, we just want to be acknowledged, and that is that people who suffer with Chronic Fatigue Syndrome should be treated with the same respect, consideration, and care as anyone else who is dealing with a chronic illness. It's not an absurd request. It is an essential freedom.

Let's pause to think as we wrap up this chapter. Do we acknowledge the suffering that persons with CFS endure? Have we advocated and educated enough? Our deeds, not our words, hold the key to the solution. The path ahead is lengthy, but collectively, we move forward gradually, step by step, toward a time when Chronic Fatigue Syndrome is acknowledged as a medical disorder deserving of our complete understanding, treatment, and, eventually, recovery.

Staying Informed on New Developments

Imagine yourself at the bank of a placid lake, listening to the soft murmur of nature imparting wisdom and mysteries. Imagine that lake now as the growing corpus of knowledge and advancement in the field of managing Chronic Fatigue Syndrome (CFS). I'm here to assist you navigate these waters as a compassionate guide on your journey to mastery over CFS, making sure you stay informed on the most recent currents and undercurrents that may influence your path to healing.

I make the claim that following the most recent advancements is not only advantageous but also necessary for people who want to effectively manage Chronic Fatigue Syndrome, dear reader. Together, let's set out to discover why this is the case and how to make it happen.

The sheer amount of active study is the first piece of supporting data in an area that is continually evolving. Novel approaches to treatment, ongoing clinical trials, and fresh perspectives on the pathogenesis of CFS are all being developed. For instance, a ground-breaking study might identify a unique biomarker for CFS early identification, which could transform the diagnostic procedure and open the door to more individualised treatment regimens.

Now, let's explore further. Think about the ramifications of this discovery. Early detection allows for quicker therapies, which may slow the progression of symptoms. This is by no means an isolated instance; a multitude of research add to the intricate picture of CFS, each having the capacity to change the terrain of available management approaches.

Of course, it's important to recognise problems and contradictory data. There are others who contend that an excess of knowledge can be disorienting and unsettling. It's critical to distinguish between sensationalised news accounts and reliable scientific studies. This is where having me as your guide really pays off, as I can assist separate the signal from the noise and point you in the direction of real, fact-based information.

I provide clarity in answer to worries about information overload. Maintaining a connection with reputable sources and scientific communities will help you make sense of the deluge of data. Furthermore, I urge my readers to interact with professional networks and patient advocacy groups, as they frequently simplify difficult information into easily understood formats for laypeople.

Testimonies from people who have maintained their knowledge and incorporated new information into their CFS management practises provide more proof. Many people who take proactive steps to improve their health report feeling more empowered, having a better understanding of their situation, and having an enhanced quality of life.

As we get to the end of this subchapter, allow me to reiterate this statement. Keeping up with the most recent findings and therapies for CFS is more than just learning new information; it's about giving yourself the power to take charge of your health, make wise decisions, and work well with your medical team.

So, how does one stay afloat in this sea of information? Here are some practical tips:

1. Make it a habit to regularly review information from reliable sources, such as patient advocacy groups, medical facilities, and CFS research journals.

2. Participate in CFS-related internet forums and social media groups, but maintain a critical mindset at all times.

3. Whenever feasible, participate in conferences, webinars, and seminars since these can offer a forum for face-to-face communication with subject matter experts.

4. Start a personal notebook where you can record new discoveries and consider how they could relate to your circumstances.

5. Talk about these advancements with your medical staff to assess their applicability and usefulness for your management strategy.

I beg you, as your loyal comrade, to navigate these seas with bravery and inquiry. Recall that acquiring knowledge is a process rather than a goal, and that mastery of CFS is attained by mastering each new fact. You can use advancement to your advantage in the fight against Chronic Fatigue Syndrome if you have an open mind and an astute eye.

Let's ride the winds of change together, sailing toward a future full of healing and optimism.

Creating Your Own Blueprint

Have you ever had a crushing sense of exhaustion that reduced you to a mere ghost of your former energetic self, as though your whole being was being drained away? If you live with chronic fatigue syndrome (CFS) all the time, you are familiar with this struggle. We've explored the terrain of comprehending CFS in the voyage through these pages, but now it's time to set your own path—a life plan created by your hands.

The difficulty we confront is not a lack of knowledge but rather applying that knowledge to create a dynamic action plan that suits your particular circumstances. A complex combination of biological, psychological, and social elements, each equally important as the other, contributes to chronic fatigue syndrome. There is no one-size-fits-all answer, so what works for one person could not work for another. This is where the issue lies.

This difficulty can turn into a crippling cycle of worsening symptoms and a reduced standard of living if ignored. But do not be alarmed; this dilemma is an opportunity to rise above the muck and create a customised plan that can successfully negotiate the CFS.

How therefore do we approach such a customised dilemma? The key to the answer is a rigorous yet adaptable technique that I have developed over many years of practise and that has helped innumerable people regain their vitality. This technique is a dynamic process of discovery, adaptation, and refining rather than a simple list of dos and don'ts.

Let's start by establishing self-awareness as the cornerstone of your plan. Begin by keeping a detailed journal of your daily routine, including your food, sleep, amount of exercise, and emotional states. This self-monitoring is the foundation upon which you may grow, not a pointless activity. Knowing what your triggers are and how you react to them will help you create a plan that works for you.

Next, make small, gradual modifications. Overhauling is frequently ineffective and overwhelming. Modest dietary changes that are durable and based on the CFS-specific nutrition guidelines can result in significant changes in energy levels. As we've spoken about, mild, progressive workouts can assist in reconditioning your body without pushing you to the brink of fatigue.

Psychological resilience and mindfulness exercises are more than just catchphrases; they are your defence against the barrage of stimuli that exacerbate chronic fatigue syndrome. And keep in mind that the importance of restorative sleep cannot be emphasised because it is the cornerstone of your recuperation.

Have you ever considered the accounts of those who came before you and survived these perilous waters? These are not only success stories but also stand-alone blueprints that demonstrate the effectiveness of a customised approach to CFS management. These stories give hope and serve as an example of the strength of tenacity and individualization.

However, what about other options? There are several alternative therapies available, such as acupuncture and herbal cures. Although they could provide some help, it's important to approach these with caution. Always check with your medical provider to be sure any alternative therapy is suitable for your particular circumstances and safe.

Imagine now how your daily life will develop as you carry out your blueprint. A midday stroll that celebrates the ability of your body to move, a substantial breakfast catered to your specific nutritional needs, and an evening of mindfulness practises that help you let go of the tension of the day.

"How can I make sure that this isn't simply another idea that goes by the wayside?" may be on your mind by now. Refinement via iteration is the solution. Your blueprint is a dynamic document that changes as you do; it is not a fixed document. You can optimise your management of CFS by fine-tuning your strategy and making required adjustments with the support of your healthcare team and yourself through regular check-ins.

Thinking back to this subchapter's conclusion, describe your perfect day when you're not constrained by chronic fatigue. Keep that picture close at hand because you can reach it. The plan you design is more than simply a blueprint; it's a statement of hope, an endorsement of your tenacity, and a first step toward a life again.

You stand at the doorway today, blueprint in hand, prepared to set off on a journey that is entirely your own. Keep in mind that a journey of a thousand miles begins with a single step. Accept the process, for it is in creating your blueprint that you will discover not just how to manage CFS, but also how to master it.

Parting Words of Wisdom

I want to take this opportunity to pause and consider the path you have travelled thus far and the one ahead of you as we come to an end of this enlightening adventure across the terrain of managing Chronic Fatigue Syndrome (CFS). We have examined the complex web of CFS together, separating the elements of holistic health, medical science, and self-care that can be woven into a fresh storey of hope and energy for you.

The knowledge I am about to impart to you is not just a summary of what you should know, but also a lighthouse to guide you through the complexities of this illness. The following observations will serve as a companion and compass for you as you navigate the ups and downs of your CFS adventure.

These parting words of wisdom condense our collective wisdom into powerful nuggets of information. Every point serves as a beacon that can light your way and give you confidence and clarity.

- Embrace Your Unique Journey
- Nurture Your Body and Mind
- Cultivate a Supportive Community
- Embrace Change with Grace
- Advocate for Your Well-being

Every person's encounter with CFS is as distinct as their fingerprint. Each of your symptoms, triggers, and treatment reactions will be unique. You must respect your unique health storey by paying close attention to the whimpers and bellows of your own body.

Realizing that their path belongs to them alone has brought comfort to many of the patients I've had the honour of guiding. This realisation is freeing and opens the door to a customised management strategy that fits their unique rhythm of life.

Use this knowledge by documenting what works and what doesn't for you in a health journal. Your strength, not your weakness, is what makes your path special.

One of the main principles of holistic medicine is the connection between the body and the mind. A symphony of wellbeing is created when one is nurtured, which might lessen the effects of CFS.

Either through diet, meditation, or moderate movement like yoga, integrated self-care practices—research and anecdotes alike extol the virtues of each one as a thread in the fabric of your well-being.

Include restorative exercise, mindful eating, and consistent relaxation techniques in your everyday routine. Together, these actions can have a calming and strengthening effect on your complete self.

Although travelling with CFS might be isolating, it doesn't have to be. Be in the company of people who listen to you, who understand you, and who will always be there for you.

Many people who have gone before you on this path have found great comfort in support groups, both online and in person, where knowledge and experiences are exchanged and friendships are encouraged.

Look for CFS support groups, participate in internet forums, or form your own support system. A community's combined knowledge and compassion can be a very potent healing force.

The one thing that is constant in life is change, and CFS management is no exception. Be ready to modify your tactics when your condition changes and new information becomes available.

For individuals who have effectively controlled their CFS throughout the years, adaptability has been essential since it has allowed them to change course and adopt fresh perspectives and techniques.

Keep up to date on the most recent information on CFS, be willing to make adjustments to your management strategy, and remember to treat yourself gently as you go through changes. The most significant person to advocate for your health is you. When it comes to loved ones or medical experts, voicing your needs is not only your right but also your duty.

I have often seen patients' lives transformed into ones of empowerment when they take ownership of their health storey and fight for the attention and treatment they are entitled to.

Learn about CFS, be aware of your patient rights, and don't be afraid to express your preferences and worries when receiving medical care.

Keep in mind that a chapter ends and a new one begins as we part ways in this book. You feel empowered and have an arsenal of newfound knowledge and tactics. More than that, though, you possess a flame of hope that, when lighted, will guide you through the worst of situations.

Is there a glimmer of optimism inside you? Let it grow, take care of it, and follow its lead.

Allow this book to serve as a reminder that you are not alone and a monument to your perseverance. We are at the cusp of a new era where overcoming CFS is a path of growth, learning, and success rather than just a possibility.

Accept change with grace, take good care of your body and mind, find comfort in your community, embrace your journey with bravery, and zealously defend your well-being. These are not just words; they represent the seeds of a life well lived, notwithstanding the difficulties brought on by chronic fatigue syndrome.

As you turn the last page, remember that this is not farewell but rather a fresh welcome to the life you are about to embark on, one that will be shaped by your inner strength, wisdom, and wellbeing rather than by CFS.

With the knowledge from these pages ingrained in your soul, dear reader, go forth and write a health and vitality storey that is all your own.

Milton Keynes UK
Ingram Content Group UK Ltd.
UKHW020644120124
435917UK00015B/533

9 798223 910015